TIMELINE of Abby's Eating Disorder— from Onset to Recovery

Abby is 14 years old (1994)

- April: Abby begins to feel the need for a greater sense of personal power, and thinking, "I'll do this my way," she derives a sense of personal achievement from obsessively controlling her weight through diet and exercise
- May: Abby discovers a fat-free cookbook and begins restricting her intake of high-calorie foods, and put herself on a regimen of extreme exercise
- June: On a summer trip to visit an aunt and cousin, together they all weigh themselves on a daily basis
- July: Abby is gone for most of the summer at camps; she loses significant weight and her menstrual cycle stops
- August: On a visit to family doctor she is told she is dangerously thin and must consume 1800 calories daily

Abby Is 15 (1995)

- August: Abby begins seeing an eating disorder specialist on an outpatient basis
- September: Now a sophomore in high school, Abby begins recording everything she eats
- October: Restricting her food and extreme measures of exercising morphs into a full-fledged case of Anorexia Nervosa
- Abby is admitted to a psychiatric facility where she stays for two weeks

Abby is 16 (1996)

- February: Abby is admitted to a treatment facility for eating disorders for a period of two months
- April: Abby's in-patient treatment program is extended because she has not gaining adequate weight
- July: A junior, Abby meets her first boyfriend; the relationship helps to anchor her, but her anorexia persists

- September: Abby has an active dating life, a waitressing job; and sinks deeper into the throes of anorexia

Abby turns 18 (1998)

- February: Abby returns to in-patient treatment—this time at a transitional living facility for adults.
- August: Abby starts college, continues waitressing, lives alone—and spirals into relapse

Abby is 20 (2000)

- June: Abby attends a Passion One Day Conference where she hears God speak to her of His love; she feels hope for permanent recovery.
- December: Abby marries a career military man—who within months is deployed

Abby is 25 (2005)

- Abby attends a Bible conference with her mother and renews her faith—which she considers a vital link to her working toward recovery in earnest

Abby is 26 (2006)

- March: Abby and her husband move yet again. Abby begins long-distance running with a running club, and spirals into a drastic relapse
- July: Abby discovers that her husband is dealing with his own addictions; their marriage begins to falter

Abby is 28 (2008)

- Abby and her husband move yet again, and buy a home. Though on the verge of divorce, her faith is instrumental in their decision to reconcile
- Abby's faith in God is strengthened as she sees His faithfulness in her marriage. She also begins to understand her body and food in a different way—as gifts of God. With the encouragement of godly friendships and family, she begins to gain weight without fear

Abby—29 to present (2009-2014)

- Abby continues a steady path of recovery. She remains happy and healthy, is married and close to her family. Her faith is center stage in her life

What Others Are Saying about This Book . . .

"This beautifully written book paints an exacting picture of anorexia, one that is sure to help legions of those suffering from this most serious and life-threatening condition." —**Amy Dardis, founder and editor of** *Haven Journal*

"This well-written book is an intimate portrayal of how anorexia claims its victim, and how it keeps one mired in deceptive claws. I believe Abby's book will help many who struggle with this." —**Dale Coleman, aunt to a family member suffering with an eating disorder**

"Thank you for writing this enthralling book, Abby. There was much I identified with, although my battle is with depression not anorexia. Your faith, particularly, encourages me that there is hope for me in my struggles, too." —**Veronica Higgins, Former Associate Professor of Sociology and Psychology at Spartanburg Methodist College in Spartanburg, Georgia**

"I found this a compelling read and hard to put down. Your book helped me to understand better how a person struggles with anorexia as well as how the Lord can help a person regain health, and renew vitality. You bring the reader into this struggle through your personal narrative and make them feel a part of it. All is important to our understanding." —**Ramsey Coutta, author of** *Longing for Godliness*

"Abby Kelly's style of writing lures you into experiencing her story with her. You will feel the struggle, the heartache, and the competitive spirit that drove her eating disorder into high gear. Her honesty, vulnerability, and conversational style make her story captivating to read. Abby makes her way out of the darkness of anorexia into the place of freedom and hope that God provides for us all." —**Kimberly Bishop, LPC, NCC, LifeWorks Resource Group**

"Abby Kelly is a freedom fighter. In *The Predatory Lies of Anorexia: A Survivor's Story*, her passion for controlling food and her body is powerfully redirected toward leading others to the truth that can set them free. I am grateful for Abby and the message she brings!" —**Constance Rhodes, founder and CEO, FINDING***balance* **and, author of** *Life Inside the 'Thin' Cage*

The Predatory Lies of
Anorexia
A Survivor's Story

Abby D. Kelly

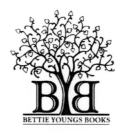

BETTIE YOUNGS BOOKS

Cover Design: Adrian Pitariu
Text Design: Jazmin Gomez
Content Editor: Barry C. Blades
Photo of the Author: Portraits International

If you are unable to order this book from your local bookseller (*Baker-Taylor* wholesalers) or online from Amazon or Barnes & Noble.com, or from *Espresso Book Machine* or, from *Read How You Want*, you may order directly from the publisher: Sales@BettieYoungsBooks.com

BETTIE YOUNGS BOOK PUBLISHERS
www.BettieYoungsBooks.com
info@BettieYoungsBooks.com

Book ISBN: 978-1-940784-17-5
Digital ISBN: 978-1-940784-18-2

Library of Congress Number Available Upon Request.

1. Kelly, Abby. 2. Bettie Youngs Book Publishers. 3. Eating Disorders. 4. Anorexia. 5. Anorexia Nervosa. 6. Extreme Dieting. 7. Self-Image. 8. Self-esteem. 9. Family Relationships. 10. Family Order. 11. Self-Awareness. 12. Psychiatric Disorders. 13. Health Issues. 14. Wellness Issues. 15. Extreme Exercise.

TABLE OF CONTENTS

ACKNOWLEDGEMENTS

This single page could prove to be the most difficult of any I've written. Where do I start? And how do I end in thanking the infinite list of people who were instrumental in helping me bring this book to life? Suffice to say, this list, is woefully incomplete.

I must thank Jesus first. A simple phrase from Revelation 12:11 was the first gust of wind in my sails as I undertook this project. *"And they have conquered [Satan] by the blood of the Lamb and by the word of their testimony."* Truly, my victory over anorexia has been solidified in this telling of my testimony.

Paul the Apostle by the will of God, says in 2 Corinthians 2:15, *"Our lives are a Christ-like fragrance rising up to God."* Thank you for allowing me to be "sweet perfume" to you in the sharing of my story.

Thank you to my family for allowing me to share their story as well; I love all of you more every day of my life. Dad and Mom, thank you for your example of love in action. To my three sisters, thank you for your willingness to love me no matter what, especially during those dark years when my eating disorder plagued our family. Dad, thank you as well for being an incomparable, patient and detailed editor. Mom, I've always called you my hero. Thank you for being my sounding board, often the amplifier of the Holy Spirit's voice. To my husband Patrick, thank you for the good years of marriage to date, and for the many we have left to share. No one in my life has challenged me the way you do. Loving you, living with you, learning beside you—all has strengthened me.

Thank you to my friends who cheered for me through this process. Dana Weatherly, there is no one on earth like you; you are indeed a sister! Chrissy Lawson, April Dean and Jackie Diana: it's been so long since I've seen any of you, but you saw me at my worst and loved me anyway. Thank you for that. Beth Petrashek, thank you for being such a heart-friend. Thanks also to my fellow scribes at *FaithWriters*, *SheLovesMagazine.com* and *HavenJournal.com*. You accepted my work and believed in my writing. I might never have started this book without you.

John Waller, thank you for writing such a life-giving song, and for granting me permission to print the lyrics to *"While I'm Waiting"* in this book. It is my honor and a privilege to share it with others.

My gratitude goes to my agent, Vanessa Grossett. You "discovered" me and convinced me that I had a story to tell, and every step along the way you prayed for me, advised me, encouraged me and promoted me. Without a doubt, I would not have written this book without your guidance and friendship.

Thank you to Bettie Youngs, my publisher and her entire team at Bettie Youngs Books. Thank you for patiently leading me through this complicated process of editing, publishing and promoting. Your expertise helped to make this book absolutely beautiful; your encouragement helped me to see the inherent value in my experience to help others. You put wings beneath my words.

Finally, I want to thank Brave, who is so much more than a dog. Our long walks helped me to think and organize my thoughts; your head on my foot made writing a less solitary endeavor; your playful devotion brings me happiness and joy.

And finally, to my readers: I pray this book helps you find meaning, purpose and value in the wonderful life God has given you.

—Much love to all, Abby

FOREWORD

Everyone has needs and wants, but imagine if yours are so deep and so strong that they lead you to self-destructive behaviors that imperil your very life. Imagine that in your profound need to be noticed, admired, and loved, you literally starve your body of the nourishment it needs to survive and thrive. Sadly, such is often the life of those afflicted with Anorexia Nervosa.

In this compelling book, Abigail Kelly courageously lays bare her seventeen-year struggle with anorexia, showing the heavy toll it took on her life and those around her.

As this book shows, Abby's ordeal with anorexia was more than a physical battle over food; more than an emotional struggle of self-image; more than a daily climb upward out of the of a mental illness. The author contends that at the core of her eating disorder, was an ongoing spiritual battle. Says the author, "The road ahead was long; my ambition to stay well, shaky. But I knew that Christ was in me. And I knew that He was going to have to do this because I wasn't sure I wanted to." At one turning point on her road to recovery, she acknowledges the power of God to strengthen her against the force of anorexia: *"I can do all things through Christ who strengthens me."* (Philippians 4:13)

This book spans a significant portion of Kelly's life from the time when she was a teenager to the present as a grown woman, and now married. In this account, she details her fifteen-year ordeal with anorexia which began when she was a teen, which she believes had origin when at the tender age of 14 she thought that if her peers saw her as thin, not only would she be more desirable, but they would envy her rigorous discipline to deny herself food and to adhere to such an extreme workout regime. In Abby's mind, that others saw her so "in control" would be a means to gaining their respect and acceptance, and she'd get from them, the attention she longed for. Restricting her food and extreme measures of exercising would morph into a full-fledged case of Anorexia Nervosa—an insidious and life-threatening disorder that would render Abby's life a living hell for many years to come.

For Abby, her numerous attempts to get well would result in periods of denial of her problem and doing whatever it took to hold on to the disorder. She wanted to be thin, and feared not being thin. The predatory nature of anorexia meant being malnourished, which led her to visit one therapist and dietician after another—and eventually, to repeated stays at inpatient treatment facilities. While therapy and therapists brought periods of insight and healing, inevitably relapse occurred, leaving Abby and her family feeling frustrated and sometimes, defeated.

For Abby, like most all who become anorexic, recovery was a long process. But recover, she did.

The Predatory Lies of Anorexia: A Survivor's Story is a compelling true life story of ever-shifting hope and despair in the life of an anorexic, and in this case, a most remarkable woman, Abby Kelly, who survived to tell her story.

The redeeming power of God's love and grace is never far away in Kelly's saga. Those who read her book will come away feeling inspired and better as a person for having been introduced to the life of this extraordinary woman and author.

—Ramsey Coutta, www.believerlife.com and author of *Longing for Godliness*

PREFACE

I have worked in the field of eating disorders for over 30 years. I've designed programs, trained residents and interns, taught classes, conducted research and practiced as a psychologist providing individual and group psychotherapy—and more. My work has been full of moments of victory—times of joy and celebration when I've been honored to share in a patient's success-filled efforts to move from illness to recovery. But there have also been times of pain, loss, and suffering when a patient lost his or her health or life from an eating disorder. It is from these experiences that I'd like to share with you a brief overview of Anorexia Nervosa.

This book is a memoir, and is not intended as a guide to treating an eating disorder. If you worry that you, or someone you know may have an eating disorder, please turn to someone you trust to help you get the professional help you need. Eating disorders are complex disorders, which are thought to have their causations in biological, psychological, and social factors. We have recently learned that Anorexia Nervosa—which was Abby's diagnosis—is genetically mediated, meaning that many of the personality and biological features of Anorexia Nervosa appear to be passed from one generation to another. With identical twins, for example, studies show a 75% correlation; with fraternal twins, the correlation drops to 12%. In other words, for a family wherein a relative suffers from an eating disorder, there is a chance that another family member will be susceptible to succumbing to an eating disorder, as well.

For an individual with this genetic vulnerability, the compulsive and relentless drive to be thin is set into motion by going on a diet. The less this person eats, rather than being hungry, the brain more or less directs the person to eat less, and without feeling hungry. The more the person exercises, the more he or she wants to exercise. Most likely this genetic vulnerability has always existed within certain people. However, it lies dormant until the right social practices move the person to engage in some behavior that triggers the onset of the illness. As with almost all diseases, genetics may make us more susceptible, but our environment and lifestyle choices either increase or decrease our chances of actually getting the disease. In our culture, dieting and excessive exercise are the "gateway behaviors" that may result in the shift from disordered eating to a full blown eating disorder in the person who has this genetic predisposition. This is why if 100 girls diet, 99 can walk away, but one (like Abby) falls victim to it.

Another biological factor that contributes to the development of Anorexia Nervosa is temperament. Temperament is the "hard wiring" we are born with. Some people have elements of all temperament traits, and thus could be described as "balanced." Anorexics tend to cluster at one end of the temperament scale, and can be characterized as "anxious" and "fearful." They tend to exhibit traits we describe as "harm avoidant, cautious, phobic of anything new, sensitive, inflexible, perfectionistic, orderly, and cognitively concrete." They also tend to be harsh self-evaluators and have an extremely high need for control.

The bad news is that the rituals of measuring, counting and calculating required to sustain anorexia, appeals to the person who likes rules and who likes to be able to predict outcome. The good news is that if the individual is able to break the demanding cycle of the illness, then these same temperament traits can be used as helpful tools in the recovery process, because they serve as powerful mitigating factors in achieving a successful outcome: recovery.

You should know that the eating disorder Abby suffered from was Anorexia Nervosa. (At the back of this book you will find more information about eating disorders, and the difference between anorexia and bulimia, and several hotlines you can turn to for help.) Abby was one of the lucky ones: she survived.

What has kept me passionate about this work in the field of eating disorders is knowing that recovery is possible. But there is no quick fix, and recovery is not an easy journey. Moving beyond any potentially life-threatening eating disorder requires diligence and hard work by both the person afflicted and his or her family. Anorexia is especially, in Abby's words, "deceptive." There are no clean "start" and "end" dates.

Initially, anorexia may provide a sense of control, but this is a deception because in reality it is a false sense of control. In reality, it does just the opposite: it convinces the person like Abby that it is there to save her, to help keep her safe, but in reality it does just the opposite. Rather than giving control with all of its demands and rules, it takes control. The person suffering is left with no freedom of choice and it is at this point that someone needs to step in and help the person suffering to find treatment to stop the deadly course of the illness.

For family, friends, and treatment providers, it is important to keep hope alive for full recovery. I believe through my many years of this work that having hope for recovery is what makes recovery possible. No one can put a time frame on recovery. Recovery is a process, not an event. It is unique to each individual and demands determination, commitment, and a willingness to explore new behaviors and to develop new ways of thinking.

Again, recovery is possible, but treatment is necessary. Anorexia Nervosa is referred to as an illness, a syndrome and a disease. anorexia results in both physical and psychological trauma. What is happening to the anorexic's body and what the anorexic is doing to his or her body, feed off each other. Untreated, this predatory form of cause and effect may eventually result in death. Some individuals can be treated in a relatively short period of time. Others are more complicated and may take years, as in the case of Abby in the story you are about to read.

Eating disorders affect both genders, all ethnic groups, and individuals of all ages. An eating disorder has more to do with how that person feels about his or herself on the inside, than what he or she looks like or what the scale says.

The recovery journey is different for different individuals. Each and every time I do a presentation on the signs of recovery, someone in the audience asks, "What makes someone choose recovery?" There are a number of answers to that question, but a prominent one is "The illness has to stop making sense." There are many difficult times for the patient and his or her loved ones during each phase of recovery, even after the symptoms are gone. It is during these most difficult times that even more insight and growth occurs. If the pain of recovery is frightening, one only need to think about the pain of NOT recovering to help make a choice for life and health.

May you find Abby's story important, and healing.
—Tamara Pryor, PhD, FAED, Clinical Director, Eating Disorder Center of Denver, www.tpryor@edcdenver.com

Dr. Tamara Pryor has worked in the field of eating disorders for the past 30 years. She spent 16 years as an Associate Professor and Director of the Eating Disorder Program at the University of Kansas School of Medicine, four years as co-director of the PATH Eating Disorders Clinic, and three years at Wichita Psychiatric Consultants as the Director of Eating Disorder Services before coming to The Eating Disorder Center of Denver. Dr. Pryor conducts research and has published articles examining personality disorders, substance abuse, compulsive behavior, sexual functioning and cognitive rigidity in the eating disordered individual. She has presented both nationally and internationally and she has authored a prevention curriculum and textbook.

Dr. Pryor is a founding member of the Eating Disorder Research Society, a Fellow of the Academy of Eating Disorders and serves on the Board of Directors of the National Eating Disorders Association. She has a MSW from Wayne State University, a MA in Rehabilitation Counseling, as well as a PhD in Psychology from Southern Illinois University. She completed a fellowship in child psychiatry and a fellowship in eating disorders at the University of Kansas School of Medicine's Department of Psychiatry and Behavioral Medicine.

INTRODUCTION

As I sort through old journals, cull memories and query friends and family, I realize how little I actually knew about my own battle with an eating disorder. Writing about it is filled with surprises still, sort of like taking a shower and discovering a birthmark that hadn't been noticed before.

In writing this book, in disclosing the predatory nature of my eating disorder, I have been raw and vulnerable—and most of all honest—as I searched for an understanding of my own life, and share my ordeal in a way that can be meaningful and useful to you.

Ultimately I would come to understand my fifteen-year ordeal as an anorexic. To aid in your understanding, anorexia begins, more or less, as a self-image issue. Wanting acceptance from others, wanting to be seen as in control and disciplined, a person sees being "thin" as a way to achieve that. Restricting the amount of food they eat, and pushing themselves with extreme exercise to work off the calories consumed, helps them to feel in control. The image they see in the mirror tells them if they are rewarded for their efforts. Unfortunately, their own efforts for the "perfect" body can lead to being dangerously malnourished.

Anorexia is different than bulimia, though both are aimed at not gaining weight. Bulimics eat large amounts of food, but force themselves to vomit soon after eating. Both are eating disorders considered mental health conditions or aberrancies in behavior based on a distorted or poor, self-image (for more insight see Appendix A at the end of this book).

As a bit of a background as to how I arrived at my own "self-image", I grew up the oldest of four girls. I remember the anthems that echoed through our home: "Abby, you're the oldest, can you please just give in this time?" or, "Be the mature one," or, "I expect more out of you."

I tried to do more. And I tried to be self-sustaining. But denying "want" does not erase it. In fact, denying "want" was counterproductive. Inside, I greedily demanded all my desires, while on the surface others observed a starving girl denying even her need to eat.

Now, in hindsight, I can clearly hear the melody of my heart all those years, the percussion to which I kept time, an inner voice that kept crying out:

I want you to want me.

I want you to think I am the smartest, the thinnest, the most beautiful.

I want you to want to be me.

I want to need nothing.

I want you to know that I am strong.

I want you to think I am the best, better than everyone else.

I want you to think I am self-disciplined.

I want all of your attention.

I want to be your favorite.

I want you to notice me.

I want you to think I am spiritual.

I want your sympathy.

I want your touch.

I want to be able to have everything I want.

I want you to tell me I can eat anything I want.

I want to be independent.

I want, I want, I want.

My "I wants" prevailed. These inner messages were so clever and tip-toed through my being in such a sneaky and perverse way that I didn't even recognize the greed. Now I recognize this greed as nothing short of a condition termed "anorexia".

An anorexic appears to be in need. The life of an anorexic is an exercise is asceticism, self-denial and ultimate self-control. For me, it took the shape of a constant ploy to get everyone else to condescend to all my demands.

So you don't think I am unnecessarily berating myself or attempting to beg pardon, let me tell you that I am needy and I do want things. But I've come to understand that all wanting is not selfishness. I have learned to ask for things, both my needs and wants. I am learning to be attentive to the needs and desires of those around me. And, I have stopped looking for others to notice and fill my emptiness.

I have found the bottomless source of gifts. I have found the unquenchable fulfillment of all my desires. I have found the solitary source for the satisfaction of all my needs: God's grace. He loves for me to come to Him hungry. However, my satisfaction and fulfillment is not the end of the game.

In his book, *The Purpose Driven Life*, Rick Warren says, *"The purpose of your life is far greater than your own personal fulfillment, or your peace of mind, or even your happiness (and I might add, your health). It's far greater than your family, your career, or even your wildest dreams and ambitions."*

Now I understand more fully his assertion.

I have discovered, in my own walk toward complete freedom from anorexia, that true recovery wasn't so much about me, my issues, my family, my illness, my health, my fitness, my bone density, my depression, my happiness, my weight or even my future, but rather, that true freedom was found only by looking away from myself and upward to my Savior and outward toward those He has called me to love. *"I lift up my eyes to the hills. From where does my help come? My help comes from the LORD, who made heaven and earth"* (Psalm 121:1-2).

Between the lines of my starvation story, I am inserting words of hope and peace that come from me, a recovered woman who is today basking in the ever-growing light of Christ's freedom for me. I pray that you see the progression, the steady resurrection of a life, and believe with all your heart that recovery is possible.

On my first day of treatment I was given a book of devotions, *Beyond the Looking Glass*, for those struggling to loose themselves from the grip of an eating disorder. In reading it, I found myself reflected in the words of others, particularly in that their admissions dimmed my own loneliness and allowed me to believe I wasn't crazy; I wasn't the only one—and I would not be stuck in the pit forever. It provided hope that I wouldn't be afflicted forever; I could get free from the stranglehold of the deceptive and predatory lies of anorexia.

In a very real way, the chapters in my book are images from my looking glass.

I hope you glean encouragement from my book. If you or a loved one is suffering from an eating disorder and looking for healing, peace and understanding, it is my sincere hope my story points you directly to Jesus. As is written in Psalm 145: 15-19: *"The eyes of all look to you, and you give them their food in due season. You open your hand; you satisfy the desire of every living thing. The Lord is righteous in all his ways and kind in all his works. The Lord is near to all who call on him, to all who call on him in truth. He fulfills the desire of those who fear him; he also hears their cry and saves them."*

—Abby Kelly, 2014

A special note to the reader:

If you or someone you care about is dealing with an eating disorder, don't go it alone, please reach out and get help. One of the predatory lies of this disease is that it's "not a big deal," and that you can get well on your own. Rarely, if ever, is this the case. Seek professional help. Asking for help is the first vital step toward recovery. Help is available. You will find more information in Appendix A at the back of this book and on the "Resources" page on my website: www.predatory-lies.com

One

The Flight

"You will never see me again!" I screamed. I knew I was running out of time as we approached the airport. "I'll die there! I'm never coming home."

"Abby, stop. You are getting yourself all worked up and we have to go inside now." My father parked the rental car in the dismal parking garage at the Remuda Ranch Center for Eating Disorders in Wickenburg, Arizona. Ignoring my great tears, he got out of the car and began to extract the suitcases, careful not to get dirt on his jeans.

Daddy always looked sharp, one more thing I hated about myself. In the last several years I had become more of a skeleton freak show than an attractive daughter he could be proud of. Now, at 14 years old, my face was gaunt and haggard and wore the look of an aging smoker. My breasts were flat and my waist curve-less, like a prepubescent boy. I wore sea-foam green sweat pants with the word "SPIRIT" in block letters down my right leg. The sweats hung around my thighs like a tent missing poles, but I liked them because I felt small inside them. A sloppy white t-shirt blaring "SPIRIT" as well, topped the ensemble.

"Abby, get out of the car."

I debated for a moment, but knew that I'd never win. The wildest of my tantrums were no match for Dad's strength, but until now, at least in the battle of wills, I had triumphed. Two days prior my parents, having cornered me in their bedroom, played their trump card.

"Abby, we've tried everything," they pleaded.

Mom spoke because I listened more calmly to her. "We've been patient while over and over you've promised to try. We are really, really worried about you." Mom's voice broke there. Dad turned and glared at my little sisters eavesdropping from the bedroom doorway. Two sets of chocolate brown eyes and one blue pair, ducked back into the hallway. Then he shut the door and stepped forward.

"You promised to gain ten pounds in two months," Dad said, his voice taut. The six-foot-four man that I once thought invincible, slouched beneath the heavy burden that his daughter was malnourished to the point of near death.

"Over a month ago, you agreed to the ultimatum that you would gain eight pounds," he declared. "You are nowhere near that. You need help and this is not a discussion. Remuda Ranch agreed to admit you, and we need to be there the day after tomorrow." Daddy turned and left the room.

I slumped to my knees on the floor. "Please, please, please, Mom! Don't send me away. I can't be gone for two months. You might as well disown me. I'll die there!"

Forty-eight hours later on February 9, 1996, in silence, Daddy and I walked into the, Oklahoma City airport. I had begged for Mom to take me. She was more compassionate and not fully convinced that inpatient treatment was the only option for my progressing eating disorder. But that was not to be.

Dad carried both suitcases; he knew all my tactics: Burn extra calories by carrying extra weight. What he didn't know was that that morning I had snuck in 500 jumping jacks and 500 sit-ups in the bathroom. I knew that all exercise would be forbidden when we reached the treatment center.

Even the flight was scary, and filled with reminders that I was frightfully thin.

"Is she okay?" the flight attendant asked as she eyed me suspiciously and then turned her gaze toward my dad. We had settled into row 17. Dad always sat in the aisle seat because it accommodated his long frame. Glancing at me, he waited for me to answer for myself. Crying had accentuated the perpetual bags beneath my eyes, now red and glaring in anger.

"Yes, she's fine," Dad promised. "May I get a Dr. Pepper? She'll have an orange juice."

As soon as the stewardess walked away, I shot Dad a look that said, "How dare you! I'll never drink those 120 calories and you can't make me."

All food represented a number to me. Dad often commented that I ate only nuts and twigs, but truthfully, I couldn't tell the difference between Styrofoam or steak. The only criteria for consumption that I was concerned with, was that it be a low value in my *Calorie Counter's*

Handbook. Flavor was a non-issue.

The plastic cup containing 120 calories arrived and I set it on the tray. I could tell the stewardess wasn't the only one peering at me from behind her glasses. Everyone stared at me these days; it made me feel uglier than I already felt. I snuggled the flimsy red airline blanket high around my neck, hoping to hide the sharp angles of my chin and my craggy, bony shoulders. I started to cry, and since crying makes my face look pudgy, I sucked in my cheeks.

"I'm freezing," I whispered—my first civil words to my dad. I knew he wasn't angry with me, but I wanted my tone to convey how furious I was at him for sending me away.

In a gesture of love, Daddy took off his casual bomber jacket and tucked it around my shoulders. Tears threatened to roll down my cheeks again.

"Do you want a section of the newspaper?" Dad flapped the pages lightly to spread the paper open. I only ever cared to read the comics, but I resented his effort to lighten the mood. He sat rigid next to me like a stoic sentry guarding his captive until he could deliver me to this place I didn't want to go.

"Is the program really sixty days?" I asked. I meant to remind Dad of how long I would really be gone.

"Sixty days is the minimum amount of time for a minor."

"What if I gain weight faster than that?"

"It's not just about your weight, Abby. That's the first important thing, but you can't survive like this much longer. You'll meet with counselors who specialize in eating disorders. You can't come home and do this all over again. Do you know what it's doing to our family? Do you have any idea how your sisters feel?"

I did have an idea, but I wished I didn't. I plucked three handwritten notes from the top of my purse—promises from my sisters that they wouldn't forget me, and that their daily lives wouldn't go on as usual without me.

A yellow envelope from Rachelle was on top, identified by her first-grade shaky penmanship, as if she paused between each letter to make sure the next one was formed perfectly. The teepee shape of the "A" in Abby was perfectly symmetrical. Both "b's" were smooth and round like bubbles, and the tail of the "y" was disproportionately long.

At the time, Rachelle was my favorite sister. The youngest, at barely six years old, she didn't understand the gravity of why I was going off to a treatment center. How I envied her innocence. I kissed the top of her head goodbye as she grinned and showed me the gap where she'd lost a tooth the night before.

"See you soon!" she said sweetly.

I hope so, I thought.

The next note was from Jennifer. I traced the outline of the single initial scrawled hastily in the middle of the plain, white envelope. Jennifer was 13 at the time, just two-and-a-half years younger than me. Jennifer fully understood what was going on, and was very angry with me for the stress I was causing our parents. Her note was brief, an indication of the stiffness that had come to define our relationship.

Kelsey, ten years old, smack in the middle between the other two sisters, was the dispassionate one. She'd folded a piece of notebook paper in thirds, no envelope. Tilting the paper, I read the single sentence from the backside: "I love you." Nothing more, but certainly nothing less. Her sideways hug at home before Daddy and I drove away was sincere, and held the full amount of emotion she was able to give.

I already ached for them. How I wanted them to miss me.

As for sitting here with Dad, I continued to rail. "Dad, this is about me! I am the one being shipped off and abandoned!" I turned to glare out the window of the plane.

"You need to stop saying that."

"It's true!"

"It is not true and you know it."

He was making an effort to keep his voice down. I, on the other hand, already knew that everyone was staring at me—the grotesque stick-figure girl—so I didn't care who heard.

"We love you. We are only doing this because we love you," Dad said, his eyes flooded with emotion. "Do you remember what the admissions person said on the phone? Even she said that your weight is at a critical place. Abby, don't you see? You have to eat!"

"I'm fine," I said and turned from his tears. It was a pointless argument, but desperation was closing in around me, pressing on my chest with each second as we drew closer and closer to our Arizona destination—the place that would take me away from my family, and away from daily habits of controlling my weight.

"I'm fine, but you don't think so because I'm making waves in your perfect, Christian family. I've become the problem child and you have to get rid of me. Daddy, don't you love me anymore?"

Leaning my head back against the too-straight headrest, I closed my eyes, determined to ignore Dad for the rest of the flight, harboring the satisfaction of having had the last word, but on the inside, my mind tossed and turned in anguish.

How on earth did I get myself into this predicament?

This is what I remember...

TWO

Fourteen—and Shrinking

"Mom, can you buy turkey next time? It's lower fat." Getting up, I shoved the claw-footed piano stool on which I'd been sitting back under the reception table in the kitchen and skipped to the bar. There I hitched my left leg up on the end barstool, standing like a pelican on one leg, a position I found quite comfortable—and provided an excellent perspective of my 14 year-old thigh. Not fat. Not yet.

A week earlier the blond skater boy I had a crush on had asked me, "How do you eat so much and still look so great? You have a perfect body."

I was 14 years old. At five-feet tall, I carried 125 pounds well, just as my genetic heritage predicted. The women in our family are not well-endowed on top and thicker in the hips. We have fine hair, brittle fingernails and several of us have double-jointed elbows. We have olive complexions, so we tan well. My hair is lighter than either of my parents, and straight. I'm of healthy, average stock. What did skater boy mean, a "perfect body"?

I shifted back to the present conversation. Mom ignored me and didn't even look up from the counter where she was slathering mayonnaise and mustard on nine slices of bread to make a whole baloney and cheese sandwich for her, Jennifer, Kelsey and me. Rachelle, the youngest, who was only four, would get a half sandwich. Lunch was always a sandwich, varying between salami, baloney and peanut butter and jelly.

I picked up a thick cookbook lying on the counter and flipped to the Appendix titled "Calories and fat in common foods." Hmmm, I'll need to nix the mayonnaise too, I thought.

"Did you get this new cookbook when you were at the lake with Ronda and Gwen?" I asked. A homeschooling mom of four girls, once a year Mom planned a long weekend with her girlfriends to recharge from it all.

"Yes. Your dad's cholesterol was high last time he visited the doctor," she replied and then added, "Ronda mentioned that she's been using that cookbook at home and the recipes are good. We won't have to change much because we eat pretty well, but I want to try and cut out a little fat for our heart health."

"These do look pretty good. Can I try making a couple?" I asked, fascinated by the idea of counting calories and controlling the fat grams I ate. Being thin would surely make others envious of me.

"Sure, pick one or two out and when we go to the store on Thursday I'll pick up the ingredients. Abby, you're old enough to really help out in the kitchen, and it's a good skill to learn early. I sure didn't know much about cooking when I was 14, but wished I did."

My first culinary attempt was low-fat Chicken Divan. Maybe it wouldn't have tasted so obviously sub-par if full-fat Chicken Divan wasn't one of my grandma's signature meals. That evening, after a brave sampling of my low-fat experiment, Dad pushed back from the table and refused seconds, "No thanks. I think I'll just have some ice cream for dessert."

"I picked out no-fat vanilla yogurt for dessert," I told him.

Jennifer made a face. "Is there any mint chocolate chip ice cream left from last week?"

"Probably. Will you pass me the chicken?" I asked, pointing at it from across the table. "I think it's pretty good. You just have to adapt your taste buds. Less fat is healthy."

The fat-free cheese sprinkled on top of the casserole had cooled and formed a brittle plastic-like sheet. To reduce the fat content even more, I had chosen not to grease the pan, so half of the chicken breast remained stuck on the pan.

Over the next couple weeks, my family vetoed nearly all the fat-free substitutes and complained bitterly. The cheese was rubbery. Fat-free butter tasted like plastic. Skim milk looked like water.

"J," Dad said, using Mom's first initial as he did most of the time when he wanted her attention, "I'm done with this fat-free experiment. I'll start swimming laps again for my heart health, but I want to enjoy what I'm eating."

Give me a break, I thought. I can do this. Apparently, I have more self-discipline than the rest of you. In fact, I can up my workouts a little, too. I'll be the thinnest, strongest one in the family.

And so it began.

I thought I was choosing self-discipline as my signature strength. While my peers honed their skills in sports, music or academics, I employed my iron-will to prove that I could be the most committed exerciser and eat the LEAST of anyone. That cookbook became my Bible from there on out as I compiled my own list of "evil" foods—everything high in calories and fat grams.

"Mom, can I go to the grocery store with you?" I hurriedly added peaches and instant rice to the bottom of my personal grocery list. "I want to pick up a few of my things."

"Seriously, Abby, why do you need YOUR things? Can't you just eat what the rest of us are eating?"

"Please, Mom. I'll pay for the things on my list."

"Okay, but you have to share if someone wants it. You are not going to label your own food in the refrigerator."

I knew no one was going to touch my waxy, fake-food choices, so I agreed.

That night Dad grilled chicken. That's safe enough. I would have volunteered to make the salad, but I wanted to keep an eye on Dad—just to make sure he did it right.

"Do you have to put that much barbecue sauce on that, Dad?" Globs of sticky, red paste dripped from the bristles of his baster—now stiff and splayed after years of painting food yummy. Mom used the same brush for putting butter on the top of her homemade bread.

I wondered if lard still lingered in the bristles. Would it come off and add calories to the chicken?

"Can you just not put any sauce on my piece? I think that brand is a little too spicy for me."

Dad shrugged and sat down beside me in our yellow and green plastic lawn chairs.

I glanced at him out of the corner of my eye. We didn't always get along, but I knew I was a lucky girl to have him as my father. More than once a friend had told me, "I wish I had your dad." When I asked why, that person would always reply, "Because he's so nice," and "your parents always act like they're so in love."

My parents grew up together in the small town of Bartlesville, Oklahoma. They went to school together and swam together on the Phillips 66 swim team. Every single day for most of their young lives, they had logged 3-5 miles in the pool. Dad has added a few pounds since his most athletic days, but he was healthy and still strong. Both mom and dad had remained active, and their affinity for physical activity rubbed off on their four daughters. Especially me. I not only exercised, but exercised all the time.

"After dinner, can we play a game of horse?" I asked. Shooting hoops is a pretty good workout.

"That sounds fun," Dad answered, "but I want to let dinner settle first."

I hate the thought of food settling heavily in my stomach.

Three

Learning New "Tricks"

Barely a month later, in June of that same year, I took a summer trip with my cousin, Angela, to Wyoming to visit my aunt and uncle, her father and stepmom. We had started planning this excursion last Christmas, long before I began monitoring my every bite. It was perfect timing, since it was a summer of freedom from the ever-watchful eye of my parents, with back-to-back trips.

Angela was fifteen already, a year older than me. We landed at the Casper, Wyoming airport late in the afternoon. I was relieved to finally be standing up, first because my rear-end was asleep and secondly because my cousin's constantly bouncing knee was driving me crazy. Hey wait, why had I never thought of that—fidgeting, moving constantly, surely burned more calories. I made a mental note to adopt this habit.

Aunt Cheryl kept a scale in the kitchen. Not the tiny counter-top kind for weighing portions of chicken and grams of pasta. At the edge of the island, right in the center of the swirly gray tile floor was a digital bathroom scale.

"I check myself every morning," she volunteered. "Depending on the number, I know what I can eat for breakfast—or, if I'm even going to eat breakfast."

Cheryl turned to Angela and then to me, "What I wouldn't give to have a body like yours again!" The compliment felt really good.

It's difficult to stare at a scale and not ask it what you weigh. So Angela and I took our turns. It became our daily practice, too. I don't remember what I weighed, but I remember that I was exactly five pounds heavier than my cousin.

"Nice, Angela," Cheryl praised. "You probably stay so thin because you run track."

I made a second mental note: *Start running.*

Angela and I talked and talked, and just before midnight, crawled beneath layers of faux fur blankets.

"I'm going to get up and run a couple miles tomorrow," she told me. "My track coach told us to run at least three times a week all summer."

"I'll go with you," I told her.

The rest of the week the three of us silently challenged each other to burn more calories, eat less food and look prettier.

I only remember tiny snap-shots of the vacation: Angela waking every morning for a run. Me pulling the skin off any chicken on my plate, and foregoing breakfast.

One week later, I flew home, alone. Angela spent all summer with her dad and stepmom. As for me, I had already learned some tricks to restrict food, and burn calories, and I was ready to employ them. All the way home, even when the drone of the plane lulled me to sleep, my right knee bounced a steady rhythm—something I would do when in the car with my parents, driving them stir-crazy with my compulsive tapping, which caused the car to shake when stopped at stoplights.

I had one week before I left for Eagle Lake Camp in Colorado. Suddenly, I was nervous.

"Mom, I'm not sure I really want to go. I'm just so tired after the trip to Wyoming and I kind of want to be home for a while."

Mom dumped my dirty clothes bag straight into the washer, added Tide, and started the washing machine.

"Sweetheart, you have to go; it's been paid for. Besides, you had so much fun last year. When you get there you won't want to come home."

"But Mom, I'm a little scared about what I'm going to eat. The mess hall isn't exactly about serving healthy food."

"What are you talking about?" she asked, turning from folding clothes. "You've never worried about that before. You're healthy and strong. You don't need to worry about what you eat!"

Thought Mom didn't share my concern, I knew the panic pinching my heart wasn't normal. I hadn't felt it before. One moment I was relaxed and looking forward to fun and friendships at camp. But when I remembered the biscuits and gravy at breakfast, corn dogs for lunch, and, spaghetti for dinner, a fear overcame me. The only solution I could think of was to prepare my body. Clearly, I'd just have to cut back a little bit before I went to camp. Gone were my days of having *Carnation Instant Breakfast, Otis Spunkmeyer* banana nut muffins and toast with butter for breakfast. In fact, gone was breakfast in general. Now my go-to choice for dinner was rice with peaches and for a mid-day snack, and gallons of water.

Eagle Lake was an expansive, sports camp in beautiful Colorado Springs. My days there were packed with hiking, canoeing and swimming. Nights were spent singing praise songs, dancing and whispering across bunk beds over the din of crickets. For two brief weeks, I didn't worry about a workout.

Jenni, my counselor, watched me closely in the mess hall. "Abby, aren't you going to eat breakfast?"

"I'm not really hungry," I lied. "But I'm sure I'll be starving by this afternoon and I'll eat a big lunch."

Jenni backed off then, but I caught her eyes on me again at lunch. Jell-O, pretzels, unsweetened iced tea. I worried she was going to lecture me later or worse, tell my parents on Friday afternoon at commencement. At dinner, I made sure to put a grilled cheese sandwich on my plate. When Jenni got up for seconds, I tipped half of my sandwich into the trash.

Two weeks flew by, and soon I was homeward bound.

* * *

"Mom, I haven't had my period this month. I wonder why." She was leaning over a monstrous book on her desk in our home-school room. Slowly, she straightened and slid her glasses off.

"Me too," she said, looking concerned. As she swiveled her chair to face me, I noticed the book on her desk, *The Family Medical Guide.*

"Abby, I want you to step on the scale. You look too thin. I can hardly believe you're the same girl who left for Wyoming this summer. I've been reading about anorexia. One of the side effects is loss of menstruation."

"What's anorexia?"

Mom stood, took my hand and led me to the master bathroom.

I loved Mom's bathroom. The tub was a huge, rich brown, marble basin. Two sinks were on either end of the long room with the tub in the middle. Both she and my dad had their own tri-paneled mirror. The only hard floor in the bathroom was in the toilet closet, and there in the back corner sat the scale, gathering dust—obviously an afterthought to my mom's way of thinking.

The toilet closet was tiny with barely enough room to sit without your knees pushing the door open. Mom dragged the scale to the edge of the carpet and stood leaning against the door to hold it open.

"Step up, Abby."

I worried what Mom would say when she saw the number if it was smaller than three weeks ago. My jean-shorts did fit looser than they had then and the cups in my bra gapped a little bit more than in prior months. I hesitated.

I wasn't really sure what I wanted the scale to read. Higher would be good and ease Mom's worry, but lower was a tantalizing option. It would mean I had figured out how to be in control of my weight, and that I could manipulate my body however I chose. How small could I get?

The number flashed.

"Abby, you've lost 20 pounds. When did this happen? How did this happen?" Mom's voice shook more from fear than anger.

I stepped off the scale and looked at her. Elated about the weight loss, I realized my plan of nearly three months was working. I was getting thin, and fooling people around me as to how much I was or wasn't eating. I didn't have to be normal or just like anyone else; I was in control of me. I was calling my own shots.

"I'm fine, Mom. Really. I'm just thinner, nothing to worry about."

Four

I Know You Love Me,
but Are You Proud of Me?

"How old are you Abby?" the doctor asked.

"I'm 14 and-a-half," I told him.

"I agree with your mom," the doctor said, his lab coat open and unable to button over his belly. I remember thinking, *You don't know anything about me. You'll say whatever she wants to hear. And I certainly don't want YOUR advice on being a healthy weight.*

"You are definitely under-weight for your age and height," he said. "You need to be eating at least 1800 calories per day."

I kicked my legs again then slid off the edge of the examining table. "Got it," I promised. In my way of thinking, he had just given me permission to count calories; I celebrated on the inside. That cookbook would come in handy again.

Mom seemed less than thrilled as we exited the doctor's office and went out into the sweltering summer sun. The visit to the doctor had not necessarily provided her with any answers as to what was wrong with me, so she still didn't know what to do.

* * *

By this time, I was also doing enormous amounts of exercise. My mom and I had been in the habit of walking around a nearby lake each morning. Now, I added to that—a jog around the lake in the afternoon, jumping jacks at night in the bathroom after everyone else went to bed, hundreds of sit-ups first thing in the morning and pushups every time I went to the bathroom.

Against his better judgment, Dad decided to engage me on my own turf. If I was going to make radical exercise a non-negotiable part of my life, then he'd join me in the middle of it and if possible, keep me from killing myself in the process.

"Abby, I signed you and me up for FreeWheel in June." Dad buttered a piece of Mom's homemade wheat bread on the plate beside his dinner of tuna tetrazzini. "It's a week-long bike ride across the State of Oklahoma."

"Seriously?" I asked. That sounded awesome! A perfect excuse to be on a grueling weeklong exercise regime—and with parental permission! "Just you and me?"

"Yep, just you and me. Hopefully we can train together some on the weekends. I was thinking this could give you a goal to work toward with your workouts. A goal with a start and an end point. But you are going to have to really eat, too."

"I will, I promise!" I was ecstatic, jubilant like a kid with a new pony. My mind jumped through the numbers: how many calories are burned on a 30-mile training ride? And of course I'll eat tons of carb: bananas count, right?

Dad and I hadn't been best-buddies for a while. Truth be known, more than the typical teenage stuff, and what must have seemed to him that I was bent on destroying my body, a wall of resentment had grown between us. But Dad was a fixer. He believed there was something he could say or do to straighten me out, something that would click in my head to get through to me, something that would convince me to eat again.

Certainly their approach to date hadn't worked: The more that he insisted I "Just eat!" the more I rebelled.

* * *

FreeWheel turned out to be my father's worst nightmare. A hectic work schedule prevented him from training sufficiently. So by sheer grit he pushed himself through four days of wind, rain and hills, he watched as his daughter over-exert herself to the point of near extinction.

"Abby, you're supposed to stop pedaling when you go downhill. Just coast and give your legs a break."

Wind rushed in my ears as our bicycles screamed down a lightly traveled section of Highway 66. This piece of rural Oklahoma was new to me though it looked like any other place in Oklahoma. Not that it wasn't scenic, because it was. In the Wichita Mountains we saw buffalo, tiny specks so far out on the plain that Dad pulled out the binoculars to make sure we weren't just admiring deer.

The yellow stripes on the side of the roads were dotted with familiar road kill: armadillo, armadillo, cat, snake, armadillo. A few Freewheelers felt spunky and stopped to prop an empty Coke bottle between the stiff paws of a decaying armadillo. Stupid creatures. I heard that they even jump up underneath cars, creaming themselves on the undercarriage—even though they'd been lucky enough to survive the wheels.

I might have taken note. I'd been lucky so far, too, that working my plan to get as thin as I could, meant that to date, I'd only lost my period and my figure. Malnourished as I was, I was still functioning. I was still in control of myself.

Freewheelers camp each night in small towns along the route. Girls Scouts and older ladies from Methodist churches pour into the campsites, serving home-cooked meals in mass to the hungry cyclists hastily pitching their tents on high school football fields or in city parks nearby.

On the third night of our trip, the ride's organizers set up a microphone on a tiny concrete slap. A dilapidated pavilion served as a stage.

"Tonight we are holding an impromptu talent show!" The announcer looked like a string bean. Her tousled hair perched like a scruffy sparrow on her head. Between her neon green shorts and hot pink cyclist's shoes, her knees peaked out, bronzed and speckled with mud.

"Anyone and everyone come show us whatcha got! Sing, play, dance, whatever, the mic will be open till eight."

The mic stood lonely and silent on the stage for at least fifteen minutes. Finally, a couple college boys did a slapstick skit and a man on a harmonica followed.

"Dad, I was thinking about going up there and singing the Star Spangled Banner."

"That's a really hard song, Abby."

"I know, but I've sung it at church. I think I can do it."

"I'm afraid you'll freeze or get embarrassed. Why don't we just watch the others tonight?"

"Come on, Dad."

"You do whatever you want to do. I just think it's a bad idea."

I wandered away from Dad. Waves of confidence were unfamiliar to me. Usually, I dwelt in the mud of self-doubt, and everyone around me seemed to confirm my propensity to fail. And here was Dad, who didn't even think I could sing the National Anthem.

My mind roiled between my ears. *My folks don't think I am smart enough to feed myself. I'm not as smart as Jennifer, nor as talented athlet- ically. I'm not even pretty enough for a boyfriend.*

Still, strange waves of courage came, swelling from my heart. This one challenge felt like a microcosm. If I could sing the National Anthem in front of hundreds of people, then I could do anything. I will validate myself on that stage. Surely a stupid, fat and worthless person wouldn't dare to stand up before strangers and sing such a difficult song.

My hands and feet made their way to the stage.

A few minutes had passed since the last gutsy performer. The weary cyclists had turned to their dinners of hotdogs, tater-tots and fresh strawberries.

The mic popped when I lifted it from the cradle. Heads turned toward me. Now or never. Dad's words echoed, "I just don't want you to embarrass yourself."

My fingers looked like tiny twigs wrapped around the microphone. I shivered, chilly even though the temperature didn't drop below 80 degrees all night long. I'd worn the same turquoise and white lined jacket every single day, along with full-length spandex leggings. Now I wore the matching blue-green wind-pants as well.

"O say can you see," I heard my own voice sing. Graciously, my brain transferred all of its anxiety to my hands leaving my voice round and clear. "By the dawn's early light." When I came to the end of the first verse, a splatter of applause began. But I launched into the last, less familiar verse: "O thus be it ever, when freemen shall stand, between their loved home and the war's desolation."

The air seemed cruelly quiet as my last note faded.

The worst part was walking away. Self-consciously, as if I suddenly had somewhere else to be, I slid the mic back into its cradle and walked off the back part of the stage. Dad found me near the merry-go-round a few minutes later.

"Abby, that was amazing! I'm so proud of you! Did you notice the National Guard guys come to attention?"

I hadn't noticed the National Guard at all. Apparently the armory was attached to the public park and the cadre had been invited to join us for dinner.

Daddy wrapped his arms around me. "I'm so proud of you," he said again. He pulled my head into his chest and tangled his fingers in my wind-ratted ponytail. I let myself sink into him; I could feel the dampness of his t-shirt on my cheek. It had been a while since I'd let him hug me. Usually he could say nothing right, simply because he was always right. And, he didn't understand me.

I didn't answer. No smart remark made its way out of my lips, though thoughts swam through my mind and I wished I could plead with him: "See, I'm good! Daddy, believe I am talented. Believe I'm strong, brave and independent. I know you love me, but are you proud of me?"

Five

Better than You

I began to see everything through the eyes of "Is it an opportunity to lose weight?" Even an opportunity to sweat fit into the plan.

I attended dozens of Jennifer's softball games, sweating on the sidelines while she pitched no-hitters and as she garnered the recognition of our entire small town. So, when my parents offered to let me attend Trinity Christian School in Stillwater for my sophomore year, which was a half an hour from our home, I didn't even consider the inconvenience it would pose for my family. I was looking forward to having classmates. And in their eyes, I would be somebody.

I was quite pleased that I'd be attending public school—though years later Jennifer would tell me that she recalled this period as difficult for her in that it was a time when—because of everyone's concern for me, that she "inherited my role of responsibility." In fact, she would recall this time as one in which my anorexia had changed the course of our family. "One of the most aggravating things to me was how much Mom and Dad catered to you," she had later written. "They were grasping at anything to make you happy, anything to bribe you to eat. They were so worried about you. Specifically, the two daily round trips to Stillwater to drop you off and pick you up at school, annoyed me. I couldn't understand why suddenly all of their efforts to teach us at home weren't good enough for you."

I felt her resentment, but at the time I didn't understand it. And maybe I didn't care.

I continued to lose weight—and as the numbers on the scale fell, the tension in our home continued to mount.

Even after a handful of doctor's visits and the threat of being forced to see a therapist, my weight loss continued through that summer. The number on the scale wasn't so much of a big deal to me, but the daily numbers of fewer calories and more minutes moving were the gauge of my success.

Now, at age 15, I began to carry a spiral notebook, small enough to fit in my back pocket or hide at the bottom of my purse. I tallied every single fat gram. By now I had memorized the caloric content of most foods and my little diary replaced the cookbook as my bible. I remember specifically the first time I logged less than 16 fat grams, then zero.

It had been an ordinary school day, but Mom had gone to meet a friend for lunch in town. As the oldest, I was responsible for making lunch for my sisters and myself. I made three grilled cheese sandwiches for my sisters. Then, complaining of an upset stomach, excused myself to my bedroom. Standing by the bathroom sink that night as I brushed my teeth, I flipped through my notebook. Excitement pulsed through me; I hadn't eaten a single fat gram all day!

I was happy about that because I felt such a sense of accomplishment. It was a personal feat, a goal met, and I was proud of myself for having such discipline.

But it was absolutely critical that I keep the notebook hidden. I knew it was abnormal to be so obsessed with food, but I just couldn't stop. And I feared that if my parents discovered the pages of cryptic equations, intentionally illegible to the average person, they would have solid proof that I was really messed up—and force me to see a doctor, or a therapist or dietician—and then I'd have to give up my rituals that kept me thin.

It felt like I was on a treadmill.

I was fast approaching newer goals of personal challenge in disciplining myself to eat less while exercising more, all the while courting my parents' concern and drawing the attention of others to get me to seek help in breaking through goals, in seeking goals for me, over my being allowed to choose my goals for me. Goals that were clearly impressing my peers. Home seemed like such a small playing field. I needed to see if I was impressive enough, pretty enough, and smart enough to compete with others at school. I wanted to be one of them, and in fact, to be a cut above them. Wanting to outdo my classmates at Trinity Christian School was an exciting challenge. And I was up for it.

Trinity Christian School was housed in Hillcrest Baptist Church. The sophomore class of 1995 was a grand total of eight students, five girls and three boys. Homeschooled up until now, I was looking forward to making my mark and establishing myself as someone worth-knowing among my classmates.

Hillcrest looked like most of the churches that I remember from my youth. A labyrinth of long hallways covered with indoor-outdoor carpeting. Coffee stains dotted the floor from the many bustling parents rushing their kids to Sunday school. Dozens of doors on each side of the hall made for great hide-and-seek—when my heart was carefree enough to play such games. At age 15, I only engaged in such activities because they burned more calories than sitting in on adult conversations.

Trinity Christian held high school classes in every room on the bottom floor of the south wing of the church. We dined in the church cafeteria and used the sanctuary for drama classes.

That fall, when our class chose to perform *Little Women* by Louisa May Alcott, I played Jo. I have no idea how I memorized my lines though; I was by this time tired most of the time, and so malnourished that my memory could hardly be counted on.

The truth is, only a handful of moments made their way into my memory of that time. I do recall lunchtime though: I loathed cafeteria food.

Given that our meals were prepared by plump cheery church ladies, they may have been more tasty than public high school lunches. But by that time, I would have rather died than eat a Sloppy Joe, or spaghetti, or grilled cheese. Ever mindful of my calorie intake, I packed my lunch: half a sandwich and carrot sticks. And, I always sat on the end of the bench.

One morning at home, I didn't have time to pack my lunch.

"Abby, we've got to go. You can eat in the cafeteria just this once."

"No, Mom. I can't. Please, please, just let me take an apple and some SnackWell cookies."

"That's not lunch, Abby. Either I'm going to start packing your lunches, or you're going to have to eat there. I'm pretty sure you haven't been eating enough."

I sealed my lips and marched to the garage. The drive to school was wet and seasonably cold for January. I hated these long winter days. With no fat on my body, my muscles railed against the cold. By evening, even my jaw felt rigid and stiff.

In my studies that day, I fretted through Oklahoma history, algebra and Spanish. Lunch was coming. What was on the menu? What was I going to do?

Ms. Wilson, the lunch lady, looked at me with surprise as I pushed my yellow tray down the line. "So you decided to try my cooking? I'm glad, Honey. You look like you could use some meat on your bones. How about an extra spoon of tots?"

I chomped my tongue to keep from screaming, "I don't eat tots! I don't want to try your food and you can't make me eat!" Instead, I smiled and drifted to my usual table.

Suddenly an idea came to me. "Hey Anna, don't we have a biology quiz next period?"

"Yes."

Rising from the table I announced, "I completely forgot until just now. I'm going to go on to class and try to study just a bit."

"Aren't you going to eat anything?" the petite and pretty Anna asked. She was a full three inches shorter than me and had shiny light brown hair and wonderful dimples. She kept Brandon, the cutest of the three boys in our class, dangling by a thread, pining for her. Anna's breasts pushed the buttons of her blouse; I was a little jealous of her curves. I'd lost every curve and cushion that had begun to blossom three years ago in my adolescent body.

"I'm not hungry really. I forgot to pack my lunch too, and I'm not a fan of tater-tots."

"Pass it this way," Brandon suggested.

"Sure." That was less obvious than throwing it all away.

Six

The In-Patient Stay

"You ARE going to get some help," my parents said again.

It was more than a threat. By now I was more than a year into what had become a textbook case of Anorexia Nervosa. My daily diet of peaches, rice and SnackWell's cookies was not going well with my mom and dad. Neither were my promises to "eat better tomorrow." At their wits end, and now realizing that I was plagued by a frightening eating disorder called anorexia, my parents called a counselor who specialized in treating eating disorders.

Everyone, but me, agreed that I need an ongoing treatment program.

The first resort was an outpatient program. I wasn't quite kicking and screaming as we pulled into the treatment parking lot, but close to it. I was there to see Kathy Hoppe, a family therapist who specialized in eating disorders. Ms. Hoppe's practice was in an office building in the heart of downtown Tulsa, Oklahoma.

An indoor marquee directed us to the reception area. The waiting room had all the familiar smell of a dentist's office: an antiseptic smell and posters of puppies and little girls smiling in fields of daisies. I noted the young model's chubby cheeks, and sucked mine in a bit.

"Hi. Can you sign-in please? Who are you here to see?" The receptionist might have been anorexic herself, or just a starving college student putting herself through school by working here.

"We're here to see Kathy Hoppe," my mom said. "My daughter's name is Abby Blades."

"Just a moment, I'll buzz her." The receptionist crossed my name off a list, punched a four-digit extension and then waited.

Mom ushered me to a couple of chairs in the corner.

"I don't want to sit," I told her and leaned back against the wall near her. I braced my right foot against the wall, locked my left knee and shook my right heel. Burn, burn, burn. Calories accumulate at lightning speed when I sit, I'm sure.

"Hi. Abby Blades?" An Amazon-sized woman appeared. "I'm Kathy Hoppe, nice to meet you. Would you like to come on back to my office?"

Ms. Hoppe had chin-length blond hair, hazel eyes and a warm smile. She wasn't overweight, but she wasn't tiny either. Anorexics notice things like that. If she had been chubby, I would have negated everything she told me on the spot. I might anyway.

"So, can you tell me a little bit about why you're here?" Kathy motioned Mom and me to a tan leather couch and then sat down across from us. She crossed her legs and picked up a notebook.

"Actually, first, let me clarify a few ground rules," she said. "Mom, you'll be here with us today, but I'd like to speak to each of you individually at the end of our session for just about five minutes. Abby, because you're a minor, I am obligated to share with your parents any information that I believe is important for your well-being. However, I will guard your privacy with the utmost discretion. I won't be calling your mom after every session."

The first meeting went pretty well. Kathy summarized our family dynamics on a large sheet of paper, noting my role as the oldest child. "Abby, you're typical of an oldest child. You have very high performance standards for yourself. So you set rigid rules and imagine that everyone is watching you constantly, expecting you to fail. Does that sound right?"

Yes, it sounded quite familiar.

Before we left that day, we had established weekly appointments reaching indefinitely into the future.

Over the course of several months Kathy pushed me to "loosen up and play more." On one memorable visit, Kathy instructed me to go down the hall to the main bathroom in the office building.

"I want you to unroll all the toilet paper" she instructed. "Spread it everywhere, have fun! Just do something crazy!"

It felt so stupid, so contrived, but I did it. I don't recall any huge sense of expansion or relief. I merely had to do what she said to be a good patient.

Seven

Feeding Tubes?

I honestly don't remember how long I saw therapist Kathy Hoppe, but I do remember that it didn't take me long to figure out how to play her. But she was smart. She seemed able to read my mind, even knowing how I felt before I knew it.

Kathy said she knew why I wouldn't eat. "Abby," she explained, slowly watching my reaction, "I think you're doing your best to control your environment. You feel overlooked and insignificant in your family. There's a lot of pressure to perform as the 'mature oldest daughter' and you struggle to live up to that. When you can't, or think you will fail, restricting your food and exercising excessively gives you some feeling of control."

She prescribed a nutritionist and instructed me to write down everything I ate. "And I don't want you to do more than 30 minutes of exercise per day."

Therapist Kathy Hoppe was stacking the deck against me; I simply had to be clever to beat her at her own game.

I loved challenges like this!

Controlling her opinion of my recovery became a new challenge, a new high. I started to be deceitful and sly about sneaking in exercise: Jumping jacks after bedtime in the bathroom in the dark; walking the long way around things, always standing and bouncing my knee with purpose and passion. But when I entered her office, a demure, contrite version of my "self" is who emerged.

"I really think we're making progress," she said one week while perusing my list of 2000 calorie-days—only about half of which was true. But my body told the real story: I continued to lose weight.

I took up jazz dance because it put a time limit on my official workouts, which placated my parents and therapist. But I needed kneepads for some of the moves because there was little padding on my bones and so they hurt when faced with the hardwood floor. One dance finished with us lying on our backs; I got bruises on my spine.

We took a class picture after our recital at the end of that semester. Our outfits were royal blue shorts and a matching midriff with black fringe all the way around. Years later someone found that picture and posted in on Facebook. When I saw the frozen image of myself, it startled me. The word "skinny" didn't come close. Nor did "scrawny" fit. My arms stuck out from the sleeveless top like sticks used for a snowman's arms. I'd decided to try a perm that summer, but my brittle hair didn't handle it well and the ends were almost transparent. It was a less-than-becoming picture—but I was the thinnest girl in the photo. That counted for something, right?

It wasn't long before the therapist, like my parents, threatened a more drastic method of treatment if I didn't start gaining weight. They mentioned things like "inpatient" and "feeding tubes."

"I'm suggesting that Abby try an inpatient program," Ms. Hoppe told my parents during a pow-wow session. "What we're doing isn't working. Abby, I'm afraid you're not being totally honest with me about what you're eating and how much you're exercising. In an inpatient program, they can monitor all the variables constantly."

I'd been found out.

Eight

Reverse Peepholes

Two weeks later, our family of six left the house under a steel-colored sky and drove mostly in silence toward Laureate, the only inpatient treatment facility for eating disorders in Oklahoma. Normally, it was a psychiatric hospital; their program for anorexics and bulimics was brand new.

I felt numb walking through the heavy sliding glass doors behind my parents. Dad dragged my small suitcase, a look of resignation on his face.

There was a ton of admission paperwork. Then, a supervising nurse led us to my room.

All the walls in the facility were dull, a lifeless shade of yellow. Fortunately, one wall had windows looking out into well-cultivated gardens with a goldfish pond. It felt like a surreal tour of a haunted house, with the nurse leading my family—her wary captives—toward the room that was to be my home for the next thirty days. Doors lined the way on every side. They locked from the outside with a reverse peephole. A three-digit number marked the address of each room.

"I need to go through your suitcase," the nurse said.

"Why?" my dad asked. "We packed according to the directions in your literature. She only has one soft-sided bag."

"Thank you for being attentive to the rules, but I need to go through it and check for anything dangerous."

Apparently, there are numerous life-threatening items that we use every day. I watched helplessly as the nurse broke the glass out of my cosmetic compacts. I felt my dignity crack, as well. She confiscated my shoelaces. Finally, she stood and then said, "Okay. You can put all of your things in that dresser over there. After that, you will need to say your goodbyes so the doctor can do your admissions checkup."

My eyes blurred and my hands shook as Mom and my sister, Jennifer, moved all my t-shirts and jeans to the dresser. Rachelle held my hand and watched in silence.

Daddy drew our family into a group hug and prayed.

I don't know what he said. My heart was saying, "Don't leave me. Do you hate me? Won't you miss me? How can you abandon me here? What's going to happen to me?"

The Eating Disorder Program at Laureate was not for me. For starters, it was as yet under-developed, and so all seven of us clients were lumped together under the category of "eating disordered patients." Our group therapy sessions included the schizophrenics, other patients on suicide watch, as well as those being treated for drug addiction. It was chaotic. One high school age guy told me about a wacky drug trip he'd taken before being admitted. Another man threatened to beat the counselor with a chair. I was terrified.

For 72 hours I was on phone restriction. But the moment I was cleared to have my first phone call, I held the receiver with a death grip.

"Mom, Dad," I shrieked, choking back tears, "please don't leave me here. I'll do anything. I don't belong here."

They must have still loved me. They came to retrieve me.

* * *

Back to the drawing board. Mom and Dad pushing, with me pushing right back—and once again in Hoppe's office listening to her say all the right things at exactly the wrong time.

Clearly, I wasn't ready to accept help.

It was a time when the family seemed to function around me. Years later, my sister, Jennifer, would clearly articulate this very fact. "There was so much tension in our home at that time," she said. "As things got worse I had a lot of feelings. I was upset that I always had to corral Kelsey and Rachelle and keep them from bothering Mom, because she was often in multi-hour conversations with you. I was upset because Mom and Dad started getting more and more stressed-out. I was annoyed that you were doing all this and at the same time, Mom and Dad were bribing you to gain weight by buying you a German Shepherd."

It was also a time when Daddy and I argued, bargained and came to a lot of temporary truces. He hoped that with the right incentive, I could be persuaded to abandon my radical dieting. "If you gain 8 pounds in the next month, you can have the Honda when you turn 16," he once promised.

"What if I can't make it?" I challenged, "The dietician suggested 10 pounds in two months. Can "we" do that?"

"Okay. Ten pounds in two months. But Abby, I'm serious. We're looking into other inpatient treatment options. If you don't meet this goal, we are going to take drastic measures."

I felt trapped. To be true to my personal agenda, without gaining the attention of my family members, I had to balance long workouts and eat a certain number of calories, which could only equal a certain number of fat grams. But my parents were offering me a different challenge. To please them, I had to perform as well, meaning doing the opposite all my anorexic tendencies.

Either way, I was a failure. If I relinquished control of my strict diet and exercise regimen, I would fail in my quest to not gain weight. If I failed to gain the agreed upon pounds, I would fail to meet the expectations of my parents. I was fifteen, and up to this point, I personally believed I had fallen short of my all the expectations my parents had of me.

Still, the battle hadn't been completely lost; I hadn't yet played all my cards!

Nine

Admit One (Only)

Nothing it seemed could break my relentless quest to be in control, to have absolute authority over acquiring the "perfect body." Translated, that meant, I wanted to be thin, thin and thin—and I could fight hunger and withstand grueling exercise regimes, like no other.

My continued weight loss had frustrated my parents and their worrying over my health and me had worn them out until they could no longer stand to have me around. An in-patient program, they decided, is the only to help fix her.

* * *

Making our decent into Phoenix Arizona, the landing gear scuffed against the tarmac as Susan, a perky Remuda staff member, was waiting to pick my father and me up at the airport.

A new chapter in my life was about to begin.

Dad swung both of my suitcases into the van, then climbed into the back seat. I climbed into the front seat, and was irritated about it. The thermometer on the dashboard read 65 degrees.

It's the middle of February, I thought absently. At least it's warm here. Susan and Dad made small talk on the short drive to The Ranch, but despite valiant efforts to stay awake, I kept dozing off. My chin dropped to my chest and my head lurched violently to the side when a bump in the road jolted me awake.

"I know she's really excited about the horses. We had a couple at home," I heard Dad say.

"Well, she won't be able to go down to the barn for at least the first week," Susan explained. "For the first week we restrict all exercise, including walking beyond the yard. It's just until we get a full medical evaluation and each patient proves that she will comply with all the rules."

After we turned off the last road, the drive on the gravel road to the main lodge seemed eternally long. No trees or leaves moved. There was no breeze either, just a blinding sun leaning toward the western horizon.

When we arrived at The Ranch, Dad pulled my bags from the van and set them on the rocky driveway. Susan took the handles.

"I'll help her carry them inside," she said. "We ask that the parents say goodbye outside instead of coming into the treatment center."

"Why?" Dad asked.

My hope that Dad would change his mind and take me home with him all but vanished.

"It's easier actually," Susan said. "When we get inside we need to start the admissions process right away. The doctor will see her and she will get checked into her room. Dinner is in less than two hours. It's less emotional if you can say goodbye out here."

Five wide sandstone steps led toward the lodge. I took the first one and turned so that I was closer to eye level with Daddy. But I couldn't look at him. Instead, I scanned the yard. It was mostly lava rock. I recalled Daddy saying once that he wouldn't mind having a rock yard; it would be less maintenance. The cactus plants looked as lonely, bleak and barren as I felt.

Fear flooded my heart and I plead in earnest: "Daddy, don't leave me. Please, please don't leave."

My usually sympathetic father kissed my forehead, drew me into his chest, whispered, "I love you," and walked away. I watched him fold his long frame back into the van where another staff member awaited, ready to drive him to the Holiday Inn for the night. The next day he would be on a 9 a.m. flight back to Oklahoma.

"Come on, Sweetheart" Susan coaxed. Our business taken care of, a motherly side of her emerged. "Chad will come get your bags; let's take you inside and get you settled in."

Dazed, I followed.

In those twenty feet to the double wooden doors that opened into the lodge, an eternity passed. We stepped into a long rustic-decorated hallway. Along the right wall, a full-length entry table held stacks of mail, each pile with a different girl's name on it. At the far end of the entryway was the nurse's station.

A small figure leaned into the window from the outside.

"Hey! Come on! It's time for evening meds! Dani, I didn't get my *Citrucel* at lunch."

The little one had a big voice for someone so small. Lavender sweat-pants hung from her waist and pooled at her ankles. I thought perhaps she was five years old, but this was an adolescent unit. No one under twelve was admitted. With a huff, this small person turned around and leaned back against the window, arms crossed.

"Oh, hi!" she greeted upon seeing me. "I'm Alicia. Are you new here?" Her friendly tone was a full octave higher than her demanding one. Her scraggly chestnut-colored hair was drawn back in a ponytail.

She moved toward me and only then did I notice the five-foot metal pole she clutched with her right hand. Dangling ten inches above her head was a large plastic bag with a tube, like an IV, filled with a clear fluid. The tube snaking down the pole was taped to her cheek just below her nose, then turned sharply upward and disappeared into her right nostril.

I'd heard about feeding tubes.

Alicia rolled the rest of the way toward me and addressed Susan. "Where are the nurses? I want my *Citrucel* or I'm not eating dinner. I haven't crapped in two days."

"I'm sure Dani will be there soon," Susan promised. "You're still 30 minutes too early."

"Whatever." Alicia turned to me. "Hi, again." She smiled a cherub smile, like the kind my youngest sister, Rachelle, gives—a smile that lights up a room and makes you feel as though you are the only person in the whole wide-world that matters.

I wondered how on earth she could seem so instantly genuine to me, a stranger—the "new girl." For a year now, I had been given sideways glances by those who first met me; I was a walking skeleton and every-one gawked as if I was a piece of angular, modern art, but Alicia wasn't fazed by my appearance.

Oh God, don't let me get a feeding tube.

Ten

A Day in the Life of a Compliant

My first visit to Remuda overlapped with Alicia's third time as a patient. An old pro, Alicia gave me a tour around the facility.

"This is the main house," she said, sweeping her right hand in an arc around her while her left steadied the pole where her feeding tube kept a life-giving vigil. "We eat in the dining room there on the left and then through that wide entryway is where we do everything else. Every morning we have Chapel in there, but during the day it's more of a den with the TV in the corner, comfy couches and board games."

My toes hung over the small step down into the den as I followed Alicia. Three telephones lined the far wall. So much for privacy when I call home.

Alicia moved on and on. Later I would marvel at what psychiatrists called her "ability to disassociate." Alicia unveiled pieces of her story a little at a time and completely without shame.

"When you've had as much therapy as I have," she told me, "nothing is personal anymore." I couldn't help but thinking that on the spectrum of maturing experiences, Alicia had lived ten lives compared to my one.

Though twelve years old, Alicia was scarcely four feet tall. She had wide round bright eyes that belied the trauma she had already experienced for one so young. Her brother had sexually molested her when she was three years old, as did her uncle and stepfather. By age five, she refused to eat—and this had dwarfed her growth. Finally, her mother did something about it.

Each time she had been to Remuda Ranch, Alicia had stayed until insurance quit paying and her parents could no longer afford it. The third time she was there on the support of an anonymous donor.

"Most of us aren't allowed much exercise," Alicia said, her voice husky from years of bulimic purging. If you're lucky enough to be allowed, three nights a week some of the girls do line-dancing in this room or watch a Richard Simmons aerobics video. I'm not allowed to, but it's almost more fun to laugh at them."

Alicia's pole wobbled as we turned the 180 degrees and went into the dining room. A serving bar, like the one in my grandma's kitchen, separated the dining room from the kitchen. Cooks were busy preparing meticulously portioned plates for forty women as well as the staff.

The scent of browning beef permeated the air.

"Tacos," Alicia said, no doubt reading my growing anxiety.

* * *

Heather came to Remuda three weeks later. Her story of sexual abuse was similar to Alicia's, except that she was thirteen and her eating disorder had only begun three months before. She was not at a dangerously low weight, but excessive purging had already torn her esophagus and her heart had begun to flutter irregularly.

Heather was never aggressive or violent toward anyone else, though she was on suicide watch from her first day at The Ranch. For some reason, she liked me right away. She said she thought I was "courageous," an admission that bolstered my own recovery. Certainly I'd be hard-pressed to be seen this way from my own sisters, who saw me, I believe, as sick, frail and shipped off. I believed that my role as big sister in my own family was another place where I had failed.

One night the nurse came to my door, tapped a few times and then shook me awake. "Abby, wake up. Honey, Susan found Heather in the bathroom with a razor blade. She is at the nurses' station now. We're making her sleep on the cot up there. But she's really upset and is asking for you."

I knelt on the floor next to Heather's cot for the next three hours— my bony knees aching from being flat against the wooden floor. For once, I wasn't the broken one. I basked in the joy of being asked for, needed. I belong here, I thought.

Everyone wants to live in a world where they feel necessary. Heather made me feel that way.

In addition to feeling useful to some of the other girls, I was determined to make a success out of the experience. I would be a "compliant" during my stay at Remuda. Besides, it seemed the only way to be discharged in a reasonable amount of time. Compliant residents were those who cleaned their plates at every meal, among other things.

In this program, regularly, each girl met individually with a dietician and a medical doctor to determine her dietary needs. Based on the diabetic exchange lists, every meal was tailored so that each girl received a precise weight of meatloaf, or exactly 1/3 of a cup of mashed potatoes, or 1/4 of a bran muffin, or five hard-boiled eggs. If a girl refused even the smallest portion of her meal, she had to drink its equivalent in Ensure. The consequences were nonnegotiable.

Dani, a tall girl with exotic eyes and high cheekbones, sat at the table once for four hours between lunch and dinner because she refused to eat her chicken nuggets. At dinnertime she was still staring at a cardboard carton of Ensure, carefully supervised by a nurse.

The calendar counted down the final days of the spring semester while I was at Remuda. So as a "Compliant," I dutifully met with the resident tutor and completed all the homework assignments forwarded to me by teachers at Trinity Christian school—and fretted about when I would be going back to school.

Compliance also meant attending twice weekly one-on-one meetings with my personal therapist, Keri. On a well-refined rotating schedule, all of the girls at Remuda participated in didactics—classes focused on the practical aspects of learning to eat again and basically, function in society. Body image and art classes rounded out our routine.

Julynn was the body image therapist. As much as I despised her workshops, I adored her. Barely five feet tall, she had blonde hair and wore it short. Her eyes were slate-gray and she wore glasses with quite unique frames. She was perfect to lead body-image classes; if any girl could imagine herself normal-sized, she would be thrilled to look just like pretty, petite Julynn.

"You're going to love body-image class this week," Karen said as she passed me on my way back from a one-on-one with the dietician. I caught a whiff of her ever-present perfume, a gift from her husband. I thought it made her smell older than she really was. Then I heard the sarcasm in her voice: "Just wait."

The first of my group walked into Julynn's office quite suspicious. Alicia was right behind me, her feeding pole sticking out of the golf cart that transported all of the girls whose health was considered too precarious to walk the grounds. I waited for her.

"Hi girls," Julynn said, grinning as she glanced up from her last minute notes. "Are you ready to work?"

"Not really," I mumbled.

"What are we doing, Julynn? I've heard rumors that it's awful," Alicia growled.

"Today we're doing body tracings." Julynn pointed to a giant roll of butcher paper in the corner.

"You're kidding, right?"

"Nope, as soon as Dani, Shelly and Jenn get here, we'll get started."

"You're going to need double-wide butcher paper for me," Alicia said, summing up what supposedly we were all believing about our own body.

"That's what this exercise is about," Julynn added. "Most women with eating disorders, and a lot who never develop eating disorders, really struggle with body dysmorphia."

"What's that?" Alicia asked.

"To be precise," Julynn said, picking up a massive book from her desk, I'll read you a definition: *"Body Dysmorphia Disorder is a type of mental illness, wherein the affected person is concerned with body image, manifested as excessive concern about and preoccupation with a perceived defect of their physical features. The person thinks he or she has a defect in either one feature or several features of their body, which causes psychological distress, which, in turn, impairs occupational or social functioning. Often BDD co-occurs with emotional depression and anxiety, social withdrawal or social isolation."*

"Okay, I admit it," I said, hoping to get out of the exercise. "I'm body dysmorphic. So can I go to the art building to scribble out some aggression instead of doing a tracing?"

"Abby, why don't you go first?" Julynn said, closing the door behind the last three girls.

I stretched out on the floor on top of the butcher paper. I knew I would fit. Julynn began to trace around my body. The room faded. All I could hear was the squeak of her black marker. It tickled between my fingers.

Julynn stood and then helped me to my feet. "Okay," she said, and then to me, "I didn't get any black marker on your clothes." She picked up my tracing and hung it on the wall.

"Now I want you to take a marker. There's the box." She pointed to a chair nearby. "Pick any color that suits your mood. I want you to write all over this picture. What thoughts or feelings come up when you look the tracing? What do you see?"

I grabbed a green marker. The therapist voice in my head, the one I was learning to imitate after so many hours of counseling, told me that green was a good sign. Instead of red—indicating anger and frustration—my choice of green might show Julynn that I was happy, even optimistic.

I stared at my outline. What to write?

I knew how this worked. A progressing compliant would write things like: healthy, normal, loved by God and unique. A more honest telling would reveal: scared, fat, strange, average, not-good-enough.

So I wrote a little of both.

I used red for a couple words, just so Julynn didn't think I was lying. Finally, I placed the markers back in the box. She smiled at me. "I'm going to give each of your tracings to your individual therapists for processing later this week," she said. "Jennifer, will you go next?"

Eleven

Sweet Sixteen

The truth in love activity was staged about the center at the halfway point of the program, basically, thirty days into an adolescent's minimum stay of sixty days. At this "half-way" point, parents, husbands, children, siblings and anyone else who played a significant role in a patient's life, were invited to The Ranch for a week of family counseling and large group therapy. In a safe and affirming environment, the goal was that patients and family members would come together to develop empathy and understanding for one another.

My family shared a week with three other families. Each was assigned a specific day for their truth in love activity. The other patients and families sat in a circle around them, with each member of the family taking a turn sharing how each felt, and telling a bit of the reality of their personal truth in the ordeal. An overall purpose of "truth in love was to express feelings lovingly and with recrimination or accusation. Each family member took his or her turn, again listening with judgment or objection. From the edges of the room, other families sat listening and learning, observing and no doubt, anxiously wondering how their own honesty would be received.

The hope was that in observing another family's dynamics they might glean insight for their own situation, and realize that they were not alone in this battle. Other daughters had lied about the food they had or hadn't consumed, about how many times they had weighed themselves each day or had a fit over things as minor as a tablespoon of mayonnaise present at a meal.

The patient's individual therapist directed that person's family conversation. Similar to a twelve-step program, each person made a list of offenses and their intent for making amends.

Throughout the first month of treatment, Keri, my personal therapist, and I discussed the family dynamics that had contributed to my eating disorder. Once a week we had conference calls with my parents. Sometimes my sister, Jennifer, was included. As our Truth in Love approached at the Center, Keri suggested that my sister Jennifer join my parents when they came to the Remuda Ranch in-patient program to visit me.

The calls home were important, and always revealing. I remember during one particular call when Keri delicately said, "I think Jenny plays a big role in all of this."

"Remember, the eating disorder isn't anyone's fault. But because Jenny and Abby are so close in age, I think it will be really helpful if she's here to be a part of this."

The therapist stressed that no one was at fault; it was simply the way we related to each other, it was just the way things were. But at the time it seemed so easy to play the victim and pin blame on someone else for making me act out through anorexic tendencies.

As I made my lists of offenses and amends to share with Mom, Dad and Jennifer, I faced the important and impossible question: *What caused me to develop an eating disorder?*

My *Truth in Love* was on Tuesday, March 12, the day after my sixteenth birthday. Dad, Mom and Jennifer flew in to Arizona late Sunday night, staying at a nearby hotel. They would come to The Ranch the next day.

I hardly slept that night in anticipation of their arrival. What if they felt "put upon" by having to come here? What if they were exasperated because my brokenness had cost them money, time and energy in needing to make special plans at this juncture of my treatment program, plus being obligated to come because the program required it? What if they didn't want to be here? What if they still didn't believe I would one day get well? Worse, what if this place couldn't "fix" me and in the end, all had been wasted—on me?

Questions, questions, questions.

What if I couldn't get this recovery thing right?

Monday morning breakfast was always a bran muffin, cottage cheese, canned peaches, peanut butter and milk. It was a relatively "safe" meal for me and satisfied my required exchanges of three bread, two meat, two fruit, two fat and one milk. The butterflies in my stomach were able to focus solely on the arrival of my family and not worry about breakfast.

Did they remember it was my birthday—my sixteenth birthday? Or because they had me and problems around for a full month, had my family forgotten me and my birthday? Maybe I was a non-issue in the Blades family by now.

"Abby, as soon as you're finished, can you come to the med window, honey?" Evelyn, my favorite nurse waved at me from the edge of the dining room.

"Am I in trouble?" I mouthed. She shook her head and disappeared back around the corner.

I liked Evelyn because she had mastered the art of being everyone's mother. She was the supreme comforter when you had to eat all of your fat exchanges in one sitting because you had declined them earlier in the day. She was the one who would rub your back in lazy circles while you cried yourself to sleep.

Evelyn was neither heavy nor thin. She always wore light purple scrubs and smelled like lavender. Everything about her was soft—from her deep black eyes to her wavy untamed hair, and even to her large capable hands. She had a daughter named Shani who was also a nurse at Remuda. Shani was still in school and didn't plan to make Remuda her career as her mother had. She was as spunky as Evelyn was maternal. Her right ear had eight piercings including the tragus, which made her appear all the more daring and edgy.

Usually, no matter who finished first, everyone at the table waited for the slowest person to suffer through her last bite. Thankfully, Shani was our table monitor that day. With a slight nod, she released me to go find out what Evelyn wanted.

And then I heard it: "Surprise!"

The shout came from in front of and behind me. Standing in the same hall where I had first entered Remuda, before the med window where I had first seen Alicia, stood both of my parents and my sister.

"Happy Birthday!" they called out in unison.

They hadn't forgotten my special day.

I buried my face in Mom's familiar jacket. All the girls, still dutifully planted in front of their plates, turned and shouted again, "Happy Birthday!"

Jenny stood next to Dad holding a heart shaped Mylar balloon.

Daddy reached to hug me next. "Happy sixteenth, kiddo," he whispered into my hair. "I love you. When you get home, we'll get your driver's license, first thing."

I pulled back and grinned at him and asked, "Really?"

"Yep! But we did bring something for you today, too."

I broke loose from Dad and threw my arms around my little sister. In those minutes, it seemed impossible that I had ever doubted my family's love for me. It seemed crazy that I might accuse these wonderful people of making me sick. Of course they loved me!

"Come on in here, Abby." Evelyn beckoned me into the dining room. "Bring your family so we can meet them!"

"I heard them say they brought you a gift!" Alicia said, bouncing lightly in her chair. For once, no one shushed her or accused her of trying to burn extra calories.

"We want to see it, too. Open it! Open it!"

I took a light blue bag from Mom's out stretched hands. No one in our family does elaborate gift-wrapping, but Mom can do a great curly-ribbon bow. I grabbed a butter knife from the table and sawed through the white ribbon. Beneath wads of crushed, voluminous tissue paper, I found a small jewelry box.

I laughed, "Is someone proposing?"

I lifted the box from its cocoon of paper and pried it open. A huge aquamarine, my birthstone, gleamed from the crease in the box.

"I bought that stone and a topaz just like it in Brazil on my last business trip," Dad said. "I had them set in identical settings, this one's for you and the topaz for your mom."

"It's gorgeous, Daddy! Thank you, thank you!"

"Oh, and we can't forget these," Mom pulled a large manila envelope from her purse. "These are all the birthday cards from your church friends, school friends, grandparents and everyone else. See, you are unforgettable!"

I heard the truth in Mom's words. For that day, I believed her.

But the lie would resurface; it was one of my grievances, or offenses, listed for the *Truth in Love* tomorrow.

I don't deserve love.

Twelve

The *Truth in* Love

Our *Truth in Love* took three hours. Blurry, mental snapshots are all that remain of that long afternoon: A yellow piece of notebook paper strewn with grievances and affirmations for each of my family members. I had the feeling of sweat-spots spreading beneath my armpits, as Dad, Mom and Jenny shared their lists with me.

I don't recall what was said. I mostly cried, because even when the truth is expressed in love, it still hurts.

After our *Truth in Love*, my family stayed for a week. I got a pass, special permission to leave The Ranch, and joined them for "normal people things." It was glorious to be "free." My family and I went to the Zoo and we played cards in their hotel room. But at the end of the week, when they flew home, my thoughts returned to discounting myself. Within hours of their departure, I believed again that they didn't want or need me. In my mind, I felt that safely out of my sight, buckled into their airplane seats, they basically said, "Whew! Glad that is over!" And, "Unfortunately, she still looks too thin. I can't imagine that she will be ready to come home in a matter of just a few more weeks."

Three weeks later, I sat in my therapist's office. I never thought this day would come; ten days away from my original discharge date.

But what if I couldn't go home?

Keri looked like a bleary watercolor painting through my tears. I never noticed how plump her cheeks were. I remember thinking, *I don't want to look like that! How am I supposed to trust a fat therapist?*

I wedged my hands between my bony buns and the seat cushion. The woven material left checkered marks on my palms. My fingers felt wooden, like tiny branches on a winter tree, brittle and cold. Keri's office was always 71 degrees, but I was so cold. My dietician, Cheryl, said that was because I had no fat for insulation; I just needed to "fill out a little."

Despite the chill, my belly burned with anxiety. My tongue was dry. It was time to call home.

I dreaded conference calls with my parents; it was terrible trying to decipher the inflection in their voices. Dad always sounded put-out or resigned. Was Mom on the edge of tears? Perhaps they'd rather be doing anything else. I was sure I was more an imposition than an inspiration.

Keri and I stared at each other across her desk. She had that aggravating steady therapist-gaze of a person fully zipped up internally, giving away no sentiments. Keri had the perfect poker face. I knew she cared about me; she had said so. But I was just one of her five patients. I was but a small part of her job.

"Barry and Janis, are you there?" Keri spoke into the speakerphone on her desk.

My parents' voices crackled across the miles from Oklahoma to Arizona. "We're here, Keri." Dad was always brief and to-the-point during conference calls.

I took a deep breath to quell my earlier sobs and suck back my tears. The taste of an abominable lunch—chicken nuggets, canned peaches and celery—clung to my taste buds. Lard seemed to be oozing through my pores; I could just feel my thighs flatten wide and fat against the seat.

"One less-healthy meal every now and then won't hurt you," Shani said, trying to placate the eight girls at her table. "I promise," she added, digging into her lunch with gusto. Like tortured prisoners, we followed suit.

"Abby, are you there?" Mom's voice was slightly warmer than Dad's.

Oh how I wished she would come rescue me. I wanted to bury my chin in her shoulder and inhale her mom-scent, a mixture of Amber Romance from Victoria's Secret and the fading fragrance of Scruples' coconut conditioner.

"Mmm-Hmm."

Keri's office smelled antiseptic. I grabbed her neon-pink *Koosh* ball and twisted my fingers through the sticky, slimy tentacles. Adult voices echoed in an alien language around me. Insurance, doctors' notes— all insignificant issues to my teenage mind. I picked the legs off of the Koosh ball and wound them around my fingers watching my fingertips turn blue.

"Abby was unable to gain the suggested three pounds since our conversation just over a week ago." Keri's announcement of my failure brought me back to reality. "Because of her slow weight gain, her treatment team is suggesting an extension of her stay here at Remuda Ranch."

Silence.

In my mind, Mom stepped out of the bedroom with the cordless phone so that she could see my dad tethered to the landline in the kitchen. He rolled his eyes and shrugged his shoulders, palms up in resignation. Mom blinked on a tear, her chin up so as to keep the tears from falling.

"Abby?"

Bile surged in my throat. As much as I wouldn't have minded being rid of lunch, I couldn't throw up. Then, they would accuse me of being bulimic and I'd never leave The Ranch.

"Whatever," I managed. "It doesn't matter what I want. You guys are calling all the shots anyway and what I think doesn't really matter."

The tension of suppressed sobs pushed tiny hiccups through my lips. I couldn't hold it back much longer.

Thirteen

The 30-Day Penalty

I failed to gain the prescribed weight. The penalty: a thirty-day extension of my time as an inpatient!

"Abby, it's for your own good," Keri said, trying to console me when we hung up from talking with my parents. "And it's only thirty days. You've already been here twice that long. It will go quickly."

"You've said that a million times about a million things," I stormed at her. "And it's always when you are telling me something I don't want to hear. My parents don't want me to come home and you know it."

"That's not true. In fact, it's expensive for you to continue to stay at Remuda. They're doing this because they love you. The chances of you relapsing, of never achieving a healthy weight are extremely high if you leave now. It would be twice as hard to eat 3,500 calories a day at home in your normal environment. By waiting a little longer and sending you home at a maintenance weight, I can be better assured that you will work your aftercare program. By the way, let's talk about that."

Keri and I mapped out a thorough aftercare program. I interviewed half a dozen therapists over the phone. Finally, I settled on Hoyt Morris, an eating disorder specialist in Edmond, Oklahoma, less than an hour from my parents' house. He also led a support group and worked with a reputable dietician.

Even though the extra month was useful in preparing me to go home, I was frustrated. My weight was the only thing holding me back. I had been compliant, done everything I was told. I had eaten all my meals, attended every therapy session and even encouraged the patients newer than me. What more did they want?

The next thirty days felt like purgatory, as if I was being punished for something I couldn't help. I went through the motions and did the same things I'd been doing for two months. My heart raced angrily when some of the girls who had arrived at the same time I did left before me. Saying goodbye to them made me wonder if I would still have friends when I got home. Once or twice I started to call a few of them, but hung up before it rang. *I'd been gone so long, they probably didn't remember me.*

Three months after I arrived at Remuda Ranch, I boarded a plane bound for Oklahoma, still one pound shy of my goal. The entire family welcomed me at the airport.

"Welcome home, Abby!" Rachelle shouted waving a sign decorated in pink and green crayon.

I spotted Jennifer first as I came down the ramp. Dad was next to her, hard to miss at his height and wearing a black and orange Ditch Witch™ ball cap.

The generous, happy reception drew the attention of everyone near our gate. Anorexic thoughts flickered in the back of my mind. *Are they doing this all for show? Do I look bloated?* Then my thoughts went to wondering what Mom was planning for dinner: Will it fit my exchanges? I banished the intrusive thoughts. Memorized phrases of truth and Scripture, my new tools of recovery, were all I had, including the Biblical principles that buoyed me: *"I am loved by God and my family. I'm beautiful just the way I am. I can do all things through Christ who strengthens me"* (Philippians 4:13).

I attended church all through my early years. When I was eight, Mom encouraged me to develop a habit of morning devotions. We memorized Scripture as a family and I even attended weekly women's Bible studies with my mom. So I was no stranger to Biblical Scripture, nor did I doubt God's power to heal. In fact, Remuda encouraged us to use familiar scriptures to combat the predatory lies of our eating disorders.

Part of the reason my parents had chosen Remuda Ranch was its Christian emphasis. While several of the patients were not Christian, and all faiths were welcome, The Ranch overtly stated that their guiding principles were based on the Bible.

Even though I had known these truths forever, I was learning to apply them personally. The road ahead was long; my ambition to stay well, still shaky.

But I knew that Christ was in me. I knew that He was going to have to do this because I still wasn't sure I wanted to.

Fourteen

The Driver's License Disaster

Three months at Remuda set me behind in all the things "normal" teenagers were doing. Though I had kept up with my studies from Trinity Christian, and was still classified as a junior, obviously I had missed out on being a "classmate." I'd missed school dances, plays and sports. Who knew how my classmates viewed my absence.

Did they think I was strange or sick?

How would they treat me?

What would we talk about?

Would they avoid me?

Added to this list of my insufficiencies is the fact that because I wasn't an "average teen," I had to celebrate my 16th birthday in a hospital!

And, now I was two months late taking my driver's test. But at least I got "re-do" on the getting to take my driver's license!

Dad had let it be known long before any of his daughters turned 16— that *NO ONE GETS HER DRIVER'S LICENSE UNTIL SHE LEARNS TO DRIVE A STANDARD TRANSMISSION VEHICLE!*

Last fall, long before I went to treatment, I had mastered the clutch, taken Driver's Education and passed the test with flying colors.

Dad remained true to his promise and drove me to take the written and practical tests the first weekend after I got home. I couldn't have been happier.

"Are you ready?" he asked.

"I hope so," I replied, but remembering I'd had a pre-license driving disaster six months ago as I tried to back the truck out of the storage shed. The passenger mirror caught on the garage doorframe, bending it backward and leaving a long scar in the paint. The kicker was that Dad had just sold the vehicle and the new owners were on their way to pick it up!

"But I'm happy to let you back out of the garage anyway," I said, remembering how awful I'd felt about the mishap.

The good sport that he was, Dad said simply, "My pleasure."

Dad put the white Honda Civic, the truck's replacement, in gear and released the emergency brake. He backed out and then got out to trade seats with me. I settled into the driver's seat and took a deep breath. I don't think I exhaled once.

Our gravel driveway was almost a quarter mile long, framed by end-to-end railroad ties. A few years earlier, I had helped Daddy lay all those railroad ties. He was a big do-it-yourselfer. His determination and ingenuity engaged my sisters and me quite a bit, and it served us well.

It was another mile or so down the main dirt road before we came to the first turn onto pavement. Highway 86 was the artery of my family's social life; it connected our small town of Perry to Stillwater. Stillwater is where we went to church, shopped at Wal-Mart, and where I had attended Trinity Christian School.

The DMV, where I would be taking my driving test, was near the airport and my friend Amy's house, so I felt comfortable having been there dozens of times before. Once there, I pulled into the parking lot, parked in front of the brick building and then followed Dad inside. Within seconds I was seated at an old-fashioned school desk facing the written portion of the test.

"That was easy!" I announced as I wiped my sweaty hands on my shorts. "How long do you think we'll have to wait to take the driving part?"

A voice from nowhere announced, "Let's go, young lady."

I turned to see a hefty, brusque woman in khaki slacks and a blue button-down that reminded me of a mechanic's uniform, except that her name wasn't embroidered on the chest. Her artificial nails were ridiculously long and painted a garish shade of blue. She glared at me impatiently and her gruffness unnerved me.

I tried to be cheery, "Hi."

She didn't smile.

I backed out of the parking lot, and driving within Amy's neighborhood on a street that I was familiar with and parallel-parked on the side of the street between two trashcans. Once I did, the woman never said a word, though she made a few indecipherable notations on a legal pad. I focused on the street and tried not to look over at her notes.

Finally, she pointed in the direction of the testing facility. I felt relieved, because it no doubt meant that I was almost done. Just a mere one hundred yards from the entrance, a tiny hill, was the only thing between the last left turn and me.

As my front tires crested the bump, I saw a pickup truck coming toward us. Quick calculations ran through my head. The speed limit is only 30 miles per hour, plenty of time. Deftly, I turned the wheel left and coasted into a parking space.

I unbuckled and stepped from the car.

"Nice job," the evaluator said routinely, and then added, "you maintained the correct speed limit and parallel parked beautifully." She still couldn't muster a smile.

My hopeful smile turned into deliriously happy grin. But she had more to say: *"However, you should have waited for that truck to pass before you turned into the testing facility. I'm going to recommend you come back in two weeks and take the test again."*

Humiliated, I accepted the piece of paper where she had written her suggestions—and on which she had scrawled a big, fat "F."

I hated to go inside the building. I knew Dad would read my face before I had a chance to explain. Fortunately, he noticed us talking and came outside.

"Mr. Blades, your daughter did very well except for one mistake," the Driver's Test Official told him. "As I told Abby, I am going to ask her to come back and test again in two weeks." With that, she went inside.

Daddy was kind enough to drive home in silence. How I hated to go home and explain to the rest of the family that I had failed.

Fifteen

Moving On, Falling Behind

My family had begun the process of moving to Stillwater while I was at Remuda Ranch. Dad had left his company job and started his own manufacturing consulting company. While my parents and I were anxious to live in a larger community, my sisters were sad to be leaving Perry.

The news of my family's search for a new house had been delicious torture, because before I was discharged, they had already chosen the house—and my sisters had divvied up the bedrooms.

My opinion didn't matter when they picked the house. Though I'm the oldest, I didn't even get to pick my room. *They really don't need me. I wasn't a part of the process at all.*

But eventually the move was complete.

I was excited to finally live in Stillwater, a big city compared to Perry. I was also looking forward to attending the public high school in the fall.

Nor could I wait to have my own bedroom for the first time at age 16. I was happy and still terribly wounded that my opinion was unnecessary for such a big decision. But it wasn't as if I didn't have enough to worry about.

Hoyt Morris, my new counselor's office, was almost an hour away, so we'd arranged for my weekly individual session to be right before the hour-and-a-half long group therapy session. That way I could avoid making two trips every week.

I'd kept a journal since I got my first locking diary for Christmas when I was eleven years old. For the first several years, the entries were newsy and light-hearted, but now Hoyt asked me to journal about my feelings and fears.

That summer was difficult. I hadn't wanted to gain weight in treatment, but I had hoped that it might free me from the constant mental anguish of counting calories and despising my body. Instead, I was as anxious as ever and even more fearful now that I had gained weight. Even now, as I read pages of my journal from that summer, it fills me with sadness—like reading about someone else's pain and being unable to help.

I'm pleased Mr. Morris asked us to keep a journal because many of the sessions were intense. I was sixteen and should have been journaling about crushes and part-time jobs. Instead, the pages all seem to say the same thing: I feel like I'm dying inside! Some entries read like this:

"Last night was a doozy. It was suggested that I raise my calories. I've lost five pounds since I got home from Remuda Ranch. When I told Mom and Dad, they flipped out.

"When was I going to be well? How good is Hoyt, the therapist? What about my weight? How long? Had I been lying?'

I felt so guilty, not to mention sad and hurt. What am I going to do? I need to call someone for support, but my excuse is, *I'm too busy*. I skip my journaling assignments sometimes too. Don't let me lose ground God!"

June 20
"Today Mom went with me to see Dr. Morris. A lot of things got settled and Mom really likes him now. I still need to gain weight, I know that, but God, I'm scared! What will five to seven pounds do to me? Don't I look okay now? I guess that's not the issue—it's when I'm healthy. I feel like such a pig."

June 23
"I feel like such a fat hog. My thighs and waist just keep growing. Then I get scared, round up when I count calories (I gave up exchanges) and then I feel like a liar and a cheater and I wonder what will happen on the scales tomorrow.

I relax and then worry alternately all the time. Help me to chill out about recovery, God. Help me to relax in my own skin, with my handicaps, and to love myself and let others love me too."

June 28
I feel so worthless. Maybe I'm misinterpreting what people mean, but I constantly hear the message, 'If you're here, I'm not!'

No one wants to be around me. Is it because of my illness? Are my handicaps and failures too vulgar?

Please help me accept love. I'm dying inside!

There are a few poems in my journal from that time. They too express the feeling of being lost in life, disconnected from people and from anything that mattered—feeling as I didn't matter.

June 30
The train just gets faster and faster.
Whoa, please slow down.
Faster, faster, clackety-clack,
Our train is racing down the track.
Once I fell off and grabbed back on,
Now, I'm painfully bouncing along.
Bumping and bruising down life's iron rails,
As we climb o're mountain, river and dale.
Won't life please stop, I want to get off!
Can't someone hear me?
Help me, I'm lost.
Which way is up? Which way is down?
God please plant my feet on solid ground.
~Abby

Cliché as it is, I felt stuck between "a rock and a hard place." In my mind, whether I recovered or died anorexic, I was a failure.

Failure and worthlessness pervaded my life.

I was the oldest daughter and yet I was failing to set a good example for my sisters.

I was the oldest but my younger sister, Jennifer, was smarter, funnier and more athletic than me.

I failed my driver's test.

I failed to gain enough weight at the Remuda Ranch treatment center, and yet, if I achieved a healthy weight and practiced normal eating and exercise habits, then I would be a failed anorexic.

Even though I'd spent much time and energy learning to "reprogram" my mind and refute the lies of anorexia, my journal made it clear I had a long way to go. The rigorous self-denial of anorexia still appealed to me and gave me a sense of power and control, even if that was only control over my own body. Anorexia was still ruling me.

"Though I'd spent much time at Remuda Ranch learning about the predatory nature of anorexia, and how to reprogram the lies of the disease to a more realistic and healthy way of thinking and being, reading my journal made it clear that anorexia was still ruling me.

Will I ever get well?

Is there no hope for me?"

By this time, most all extended family and friends knew me as anorexic—and recognized me as a fanatical exerciser and the one who never ate in social situations.

But while I failed them because I wasn't a "healthy teen," I wasn't prepared to fail my eating disorder just yet.

Sixteen

The Boyfriend

Writing, whether journaling or letters, has been most effective for me in communicating my feelings with others. My sister Jennifer wrote this letter explaining how she felt during my eating disorder. She has sharp memories of my years with anorexia, more than either of my other sisters. It's my sense that because of our closeness in age, she experienced the fallout most acutely.

"It baffled me that you would talk about having to "work, work, work" when there was no reason you had to have a job. Honestly I knew it was because you didn't want to be at home. I remember the parade of boyfriends you had and that just baffled me. The girls on the swim team were shocked at what a prude I was. When they found out we were sisters, it made me feel like I didn't know who you were at all."
~Jennifer, 2013

Jenny was caught between fear for me and fury with me. To her it seemed like I was ungrateful and rebellious. She felt forced into the role of "big sister" to Kelsey and Rachelle. I was too self-consumed with my pursuit of perfection and identity to consider whether I was expressing love to my family.

Three months after I left Remuda, now 16 years, 5 months old, I started my junior year at Stillwater High School. I didn't experience the system shock that everyone feared for a long-term home-schooled student. The very first day, I caught the eye of a cute boy and set the tone for my high school experience-boyfriends and work. Between my part-time job as a hostess at Red Lobster and the challenge of proving to myself that I was pretty and desirable to the opposite sex, I spent no time with my family.

Jennifer was right, I did anything that kept me away from home and my parents out of my business.

Chad and I had first met at our parents' high school reunion. The event was held at Kitty Land, a small amusement park in Bartlesville, Oklahoma. It was a late summer evening and the scents of barbecue and cotton candy hung heavy in the air. I felt a little out of place, unable to bring myself to fill a paper plate with picnic food, sit on the grass and talk with the adults, and too old to ride the rides with the youngest kids.

Chad was just like his dad: sandy blond hair, light brown eyes and big hands. I was an inexperienced flirt, but Chad had it down pat. After the briefest of introductions by our parents, he grabbed my elbow and suggested we walk around the park. Before I knew it, we were holding hands.

"You'll love Stillwater High," he told me. "I'll get you into choral. Mr. Mason has been our director for years and he's really talented. In fact, I'm in a quartet with his son and a couple other guys. We're pretty good; we get to perform around town at special events."

Chad had a knack for building his own self-esteem. "Friday is registration at SHS. I don't really have to go. I did it early, but if you want I'll meet you there. I can take you around and introduce you to most of the teachers and some of the other kids that will be there, too."

On registration day, I don't remember a single teacher's face and I couldn't keep up with the paperwork for numerous classes, signatures and what seemed like ten pounds of books. But I do remember Chad's escort. Afterwards he walked me to my car.

"Hey, I know this is fast," Chad began. "But, I think you're beautiful." He was one for flattery.

"A week from Monday, all the other guys are going to get a shot at you. So, I'm taking a head start. Will you go out with me?"

Wow, that was easy, I thought. Though not at all confident, I told him "Yes!"

Chad was amazing. Because of him, I was at once popular at Stillwater High School. Starting with a boyfriend put me ahead of all the seasoned public school girls who had dumped their boyfriends over the summer in favor of older lifeguards.

Every day at lunch I tagged along with Chad and his musical buddies to wherever they chose for lunch. On most days Chad voted for my favorite place, The Bagel Shop.

There I knew I could eat a plain jalapeño bagel and a bag of pretzels for 400 calories. With enough Diet Pepsi, I felt full for the rest of the day.

Most of my new friends didn't know that I'd spent the final part of my sophomore year at an inpatient facility for the mentally ill—as eating disorders are categorized. A few commented once or twice about my strange eating habits, like dipping each bite of my jalapeño bagel in a mountain of salt or the fact that I could drink forty ounces a day of gas station coffee. But most actually admired my commitment to hit the gym everyday even though I didn't play any sports. I was enviably skinny to the girls and "fresh meat" to the boys on our high school campus. Few knew the anguish I suffered everyday trying to stay "perfect."

Some days I stayed after school to watch Chad rehearse with the quartet. They were fabulous and my girlish heart raced with pride and swooned with admiration for this talented boy who "loved" me. On those days, he drove me home since my house was only half a mile away and on his way home.

In retrospect, I see that most everything we did was Chad's idea, Chad's choice, Chad's hobby, and Chad's friends. He was an easy guy to hide behind. He was welcomed everywhere and everyone loved him. In his wake, the waters of popularity were calm.

To be fair, I owe Chad for my smooth transition into cliquish Stillwater High. But with him I learned early that I had to give up something to receive the love I craved. Fortunately, with him, the cost was low.

With the start of football season comes high speed flirting and hooking up at a high school. I had chills arriving to games early with Chad. The quartet usually performed the National Anthem before the game. They were flawless and I saw Chad wink at me from the sidelines.

Chad always stayed to the bitter end. His socialite status demanded that he talk to everyone—and their parents, too. Finally, we clambered down the bleachers at nearly 10:00 pm. My curfew was 11:30, plenty of time.

Chad drove slowly up North Washington Street, the last street before my parents' neighborhood. My heart clung to my ribs when he braked and veered right into Will Roger's Elementary School parking lot. My only fear was halitosis—bad breath, which was yet another bad side-effect of anorexia. I knew what was coming.

In an instant, Chad was out of the truck and opening my side of the door. I slid across the seat and like Cinderella, took his hand and stepped delicately out of the filthy pickup. We hopped onto the tailgate leaving prints of our rear-ends in the dirty film. He put his arm around my waist really low and then his hand on my face.

I remember sensations, nerves standing on end in every place he touched, but I don't remember his face or his words—until our lips met. I could hear Kenny Chesney crooning from the radio as Chad's lips felt soft and too wet. I wasn't sure I liked swapping spit, but I had to stick it out; this was what every high school girl lives for, right?

I tilted my head right, hoping to do the movie-style head twisty thing, but Chad tilted his head the same way. Quick corrections sent us both the same direction to the other side. Suddenly, I felt a tap against my lips, something even wetter. I pulled back sharply, fighting the urge to cough, wipe my mouth or spit.

Chad came in again for another pass, obviously unaware of my distress. Desperately I tried to be a good sport and not jerk away, but I staunchly sealed my lips. I felt him licking my lips now. Slowly, it seemed to dawn on him that I didn't know what French kissing was, though I was thinking I probably wasn't into it anyway. He pulled back and slid off the tailgate. He helped me down and opened my door.

"You could use some practice," he said.

Two weeks later, Chad was kissing someone else. But I'd gotten my feet wet, and there were a lot more fish in the sea.

Seventeen

Boys Boys Boys

The academics were less than challenging for me. Home schooling had moved me well ahead of my classmates at school—which was very good news in that it left me with plenty of time for dating.

At the beginning of my junior year, I was pegged "Ice Princess." I remember hearing snippets of gossip about me in the halls.

"I'd tap that" was a phrase I hadn't heard up to now, so I had to ask a few friends to clarify what it meant. I learned that it meant something to the effect, "I'd have sex with her." It was probably more bravado than anything, but I was embarrassed even hearing it.

For the next two years at Stillwater High School, I maintained a weight that kept my parents and Dr. Morris satisfied. And at least Dr. Morris wasn't advocating inpatient therapy again. But though I kept good grades and did well at my job waiting tables at Red Lobster, my parents continued to fret.

"Abby, I wish you'd relax a little; you have terrible bags under your eyes," Mom said, one day as she stood across the kitchen island, arms crossed, gaze stern. "I know you are tired and are not taking care of your body."

Coming in from the garage, Dad had heard her comment, and added, "Why don't you stay home for dinner tonight?"

"Can't." I popped a grape into my mouth, making my point wordlessly—I am eating, so you can't complain. Besides, I'll grab something at Red Lobster after my shift. You know I get a free shift meal."

"The problem is I don't know if I believe you," Mom said, and then left the room before I could argue my case.

My parents were right, though. I wasn't being honest with them about how much or when I ate. I was also sneaking in workouts when they thought I was working at the restaurant.

Jennifer had been right in her letter when she accused me of not wanting to be at home. It was easier not to be home. At home, everyone knew my habits surrounding restricting my food intake and my penchant for extreme amounts of exercise. At home, everyone watched me—constantly. At home, my anorexia and I were constantly scrutinized.

But I was a little scared for myself, too, because my weight continued to drop. My jeans were getting looser, and yet, I was skipping class to go to the gym and obsessively counting calories. I was walking a dangerous line. If I didn't put on some weight, my parents would send me back to treatment. Or what if I really did die?

At the same time, I was scared to be well—because getting "well" meant that I'd be putting on weight—and I genuinely wanted to be thin. What if gaining weight in order to be well, things got out of hand; what if I ended up fat? Who would I be then? Being thin was my identity... and I liked it. Everyone knew me as the thinnest girl, the one with the strongest will. If I allowed myself to gain weight it would prove that I was weak. At least with anorexia I had an identity, I wasn't just one of the crowd.

And of course I had to continue to lie to my family, and as well, to pacify them that I was watching out for myself. And, I had to get snarky when I needed to, to basically try to keep them at bay so that my anorexia could continue the love/hate relationship we had going on.

I was scared that if my family knew I was still sick, they would force me to go back to treatment.

I didn't know what I wanted, but I didn't know how long I could hold on—lying to everyone while secretly rooting to keep my life as an anorexic alive and well—and without anyone finding out that this was what I wanted.

If only I lived by myself—then I could do all this without having to work so hard at controlling everyone!

I might have denied my hunger for food, but now in high school, I had an insatiable appetite for boys. Already I had a big appetite for approval, appreciation and acceptance from my classmates, but as for the boys—I wanted to be thought of as irresistible.

And so I worked to bring that about. Unfortunately, most of the attention from boys was fleeting at best. They took what they wanted, as much as I would give physically, flattered me as they indulged and then left as quickly as they came. But in as much as I didn't want them to come into and go out of life as quickly as they did, the truth is, I usually tired of them first. I wasn't interested in them as people or in having a long-term relationship with them. I merely needed them to validate me. I was consumed with my relationship with anorexia.

One after another.

After Chad there was Saul—his best friend. Chad didn't care. I think I'd been more of a social experiment for him—the dating a girl fresh from the protective shelter of home schooling.

Later I dated Josh but only for a couple of weeks. What flattery that was! He was hot, on the baseball team and the quiet kind of popular. Rumors flew through the halls of Stillwater High long before he asked me out, that he was interested in me.

"Did you know Josh likes you? He's gorgeous; you're so lucky!" the girls told me.

And with the flattery, came a warning, "Abby, all he really wants is sex. Josh has a reputation that way. You can't trust him; he's cheated on everyone he's ever dated."

Josh flaunted an air of superiority, taking ego to a whole new level. I was lucky to be dating him, he insinuated. His indifference made me want him to want me all the more.

Around Christmas time, after Josh and I had been dating for about a month, I took him home to meet my family. Unfortunately he made a bad impression. He showed up on the front porch in faded blue jeans with the back left pocket ripped out, exposing his red, plaid boxers. My parents and sisters disapproved from the very moment they saw him.

Josh is the benchmark in my timeline when I became willing to go further physically. Though not ready to surrender my virginity, there was little I wouldn't do.

At first, I balked when he pushed too hard for or wanted to go too far, but by the time we broke up, less than three months after we'd considered ourselves a couple, I found myself more willing to do whatever it took to satisfy my craving for affirmation that I was desirable, "hot," loving—and lovely.

Next came Chris. By the time I dated Chris, I had a string of make-out partners on the side. Matt, Steven, Ryan, Brian, Sean, John—and a few names I don't remember. Matt had told me I was the best kisser ever. I balanced on a tightrope between tease and slut, ice queen and easy.

Then I met Buck.

Buck was a cook at Red Lobster where I had been waitressing for a little over a year. He was 21; I was nearly 17. We winked at each other over the warming oven in the kitchen. The flirting was casual and we rarely even spoke except to say "Hi." Finally, one night we got off work about the same time and he walked me to my car. In the course of one conversation, he convinced me to come to his apartment later that night. I went home and pretended to go to bed as usual. At eleven, when I knew my parents were sound asleep, I snuck out of the house, pushed my standard transmission Honda into the street and drove to his apartment. Excited to be with him, my nerves tingled on an adrenaline high.

He met me at the door.

"You're beautiful," he said and I knew he meant it.

Buck pushed the hair back from my cheeks, cupped my face and kissed me lightly. Then he pulled me inside.

George Straight crooned the most perfect words: "In all this world, you'll never find, a love as true, as mine."

Buck had prepared for me. Six creamy white candles lit the sparsely furnished room. Unfortunately the room smelled a little stale, and the dining bar, which separated the living room from the kitchen, needed a good sponge.

"Come here," he said, oblivious to everything but me.

Buck was so gentle. He lay me down on my back on his mattress, and knelt over me.

I wanted it. Oh, how I wanted it. I wanted to make him happy. I wanted to impress him with my kisses, my sultry tone, but when he began to unbutton my pants, I didn't want that.

"I'm sorry, I can't. I have to go. I'm sorry," I said, scrambling to my feet. I grabbed my keys and fled down the stairwell, back to my car and reversed the process. I tiptoed back into the safety of my parents' home and slid between the covers of my sheets.

I had gone and returned within an hour.

Still, Buck had won my heart that night.

He called again, and he continued to flirt with me at the restaurant. He hadn't forgotten about me when I said "no." So, I brought him home to meet my parents. He charmed them, too. Other than our age difference, Buck appeared to be everything a parent could want for their daughter. So I bid adieu to the high school dating scene, and Buck became my "guy."

The relationship was sweet. Here was a guy who actually "saw" me—and treated me as though I was "special." What I wanted meant something to him. Buck never pushed for more than I didn't willingly give.

In time, he became not only my boyfriend, but seen as a part of our family. He'd make Mother's Day brunch for my mom; he attended church with our family; he'd help with chores such as cleaning our pool. He even attended functions such as my sisters' sporting events.

Because of Buck, I stopped my attempts to solicit yet a next victim to feed my ego its dose of admiration. Buck became enough. His admiration was "enough." And because my family liked him, and that he liked my family, it made everything less complicated and easier to be at home. And, it made it easier to gain some distance between me the "sick, skinny kid they knew me to be," and helped them to see a more "normal" teen daughter.

Six months from the day Buck and I met, he asked me to marry him. He followed protocol, asking first my dad, and then bought a ring.

But Daddy didn't say yes, and in fact, told Buck to wait "indefinitely."

But at least I was loved. And felt loved. Buck had become "my love."

As did God.

I suddenly felt anew. God's love began to move in my heart during those waiting months. And this may have been the dawning for me, that I had a future outside the approval of others. Maybe I could be okay just by myself. Suddenly, I didn't want to know what "the rest of my life" looked like.

I broke up with Buck.

It shattered him and there were dozens of tearful messages on the answering machine.

Eighteen

The Guardianship

With my eighteenth birthday fast approaching and Remuda Ranch almost two years in the distant past, things were worse than they'd ever been.

Since Remuda Ranch, my weight had plummeted making everyone around me scared for me—and threatening to send me back to an in-patient treatment program.

I was scared for me also, but for a different reason: I was scared that I'd be forced to get well—and that would mean I'd gain weight.

So far I had balanced controlling others to leave me alone, while still restricting the amount of food I ate, doing extreme exercise and obsessively counting calories. This made it easier to lay low and not subject myself to everyone always looking in on how much I ate; I distanced myself from family—as well as everyone else who cared about me.

While I was concerned because my extreme weight loss was evident to me too, I was concerned that if I started eating or stopped exercising, then I'd gain weight.

I'd long ago became an addict to the disease of anorexia, and was scared that it would be taken away from me. I had to make sure I wasn't forced to go back to treatment.

I didn't know how long I could hold on.

Daddy and I were back to bargaining, primarily because in over a year, I had still not reached the weight goal that Remuda set for me.

"Abby, you need to reach 118 pounds by the New Year," Dad said. "If you don't, we are going to seriously look into inpatient treatment options again."

Fall had come and it was one of the last long nights of summer. The goblins and ghosts of Halloween began popping up in stores everywhere. It had been almost exactly three years since my dad and I had a similar conversation.

Now we stood in the empty garage, shedding mud boots and coveralls after feeding the three dogs, I leaned against the wall so as to pull a stubborn boot over my heel.

"But," I stopped quickly; Dad hated to be interrupted.

"But, if you reach 118," he hurried to finish the thought, "and maintain it through graduation in May, you can have the Honda free and clear."

Images of car keys danced in my head, but I had a long way to go to take him up on the bribe.

"There's another part to this deal," Dad continued. "Let's go inside. I want your mom to be a part of this conversation."

In the kitchen, Dad pulled out a chair at the dining table and motioned for me to sit down. "J," he called for my mom. "Let's just get this over with now."

Uh-oh.

We sat around the dinner table. I splayed my palms flat and analyzed the chipped pink polish. My eyes traveled up my arms tracing the crochet pattern on my oversized sweater. I liked wearing winter clothes; there was less of my body to see, less of my body to criticize.

"We have a court date tomorrow," Dad began.

"What for?"

"Your mom and I have requested legal guardianship of your medical care. You'll be 18 in March and you haven't demonstrated the ability to care for your own body like an adult."

"Are you serious?" My voice rose in rage. The audacity! I was 17 and it was high time that people let me have a life of my own.

"We can do this one of two ways," Mom said. "First, you can go with us tomorrow at 4 o'clock, after school, and agree to the terms of our petition. But, if you won't, we'll have to appeal and this will be a very complicated process. It's up to you."

I knew well the voices of the proverbial angel and demon perched on my shoulder, each trying to out-yell the other. Lately, the demon had been viciously loud, screaming at me night and day.

Just last night in my journal I had confessed my own hopelessness.

All this time, and still, I didn't want to travel this same road all over again, but I didn't know how to turn around.

December 29

I feel like the only person in the whole world. Surrounded by people, friends and family who say they care, but somehow I can't believe them. I am feeling so lonely, inadequate, unworthy, unmotivated, small, despicable, rejected and friendless. I am so tired. I am nowhere near a "successful" weight. I feel ugly, sick and jobless as a result, and simply hopeless.

Should I end it all? Wouldn't that be easier? Snap my neck, pull a trigger, stab a knife, swallow pills. No more pain. But something won't let me. What is it? God, is it you?

I know it's You; You love me. I feel like I'm on the edge of some breakthrough to being at peace in you. But I can't actually get there. All the tools are in my hands, plans in my head and I still battle myself every day and never win!

I feel like I'm fighting against everyone simply for survival.

Help me please!

—Abby

As I poured out my prayer that night, I heard Jesus insisting, "Abby, I want to fight for you. Please quit, lay down your sword. I've already won this battle."

It was a soft voice, the whisper behind the tyrannical rush of thoughts.

* * *

I came back to the present. "Okay," I said, tilting my chair backwards on its hind legs, just like I'd been doing—and instructed not to do—since I was a little girl. "I'll agree to it."

Suddenly, a sweet peace swept over me. I dropped the legs of my chair, leaned over and buried my face in my arms.

My very soul was tired of this fight. The stakes were too high. A part of me was even ready to return to Remuda that very night.

Truth is, I couldn't survive in this real life.

Nineteen

Happy Birthday—and Welcome Back

February 26

Who am I to define "perfect" to my perfect Creator?

That's all I've ever wanted: To design the perfect body. I just want to do something perfect. And here I am stressed to the max, hoping to become something I can't even recognize.

But I do see perfection in others—my dad's job, my sisters' athletics. Why can't I be a good anorexic? All this trying to be perfect has gotten me in trouble with my parents, so I try harder at my job, promotions, school, grades, chores, gifts, spirituality, time at home, being productive, buying my own car, writing, cleaning, walking the dog, watching my money, praying for my family.

But I can't let go of anorexia.

Why? Because it's MINE, MINE, MINE! I want it! I feel like a baby being weaned off a pacifier. I am screaming, *"Give it back, it makes me happy. It gives me individuality. It's my advantage, my goal, my personal challenge. It's my way to prove my strength."*

I'm not crazy; I know what I'm doing. Please, why can't everyone just leave me alone?

Love me gently because I'm your daughter, not because I'm sick (you think) and don't give up on me. Just love and hold me and please stop with the demands. Just shut up!

* * *

The next month, at the beginning of March, just before I turned 18, my parents persuaded me to go back Remuda. I had spent my 16th birthday there; now I would spend my 18th birthday at The Ranch.

Once again, it was required to stay at The Ranch for a minimum of sixty days. Initially, my stay was at the main lodge, exactly where I'd been two years before. It was humbling to see some of the same therapists and nurses again. I felt like I'd failed them. A few days after, my stay moved from the main campus to Chandler, Arizona because I became a legal adult. This was Remuda's partial-care program.

I wasn't really sure how I ended up at Remuda Ranch again. Had it been my decision or my parents? It was their idea and at their insistence, but I hadn't fought them this time.

Dad had broached the subject late one Tuesday evening.

"Abby, we've contacted Remuda Ranch because your mom and I think you need intensive treatment again. Tomorrow after school, the admission's counselor is going to call and interview you. If they agree that you need to be inpatient again, they have already informed me that they have space. You need to be prepared to leave for Arizona on Friday."

I cried, but I didn't scream. I sobbed, but I didn't know why.

"Ok," I managed to whisper.

I was torn. The idea of going back to Remuda terrified me. Of course they would force me to gain weight again. At the same time I didn't want to live this way anymore. I was tired of hiding from and lying to my parents. I was tired of avoiding every meal and dreading the holidays. I was tired of being cold all the time and tired of the constant chaotic thoughts about exercise and calories.

This was the crucible. Either I must trust what others were telling me—that I would be okay when I gained weight, that I could be happy again, or I needed to give up now and die. Anorexia was making me miserable and life wasn't worth living this way.

March 17

It's a couple of weeks later and guess where I am? I am at Remuda Ranch, this time at their center in Chandler!

I flew up here alone. I am living unsupervised, but I am so ready, I think, to get well.

I want to kick this. Right now, I feel so good. God, help me to remember this feeling even when I am down. You are always there. Help me to be comfortable around the people who love me. Teach me to trust You; I know I can. I need you so much, Lord. Never let me go, please! Provide for me everything that I need. I love you, Lord, and I want to let this go. Please, help me.

Abby

* * *

Chandler, also called "The Cul-de-sac," was a cozy little circle of seven homes. Each housed four or five women. Chandler was designed to provide a middle step, a cautious introduction to the real world for fragile, barely recovered eating disordered patients.

Maybe that's what I had missed the first time; at least it was what I desperately needed this time.

How do I live like an adult? How do I feed myself?

Teri was my roommate. The first time I met her, she was wearing a baseball hat with the letters OSU.

"Are you from Oklahoma?" I asked. "I'm going to Oklahoma State next semester when I get out of here."

Teri flopped onto her bed, rumpling the covers, and didn't straighten them when she got back up.

"Nope, I'm going to Ohio State. I hadn't noticed that before—same initials; how cool!"

Our room was small, barely wide enough for two twin beds. Both headboards butted up to the same wall, with a cheery window between them. Teri slid the window open, letting the yellow gingham curtains flutter.

"I'm so, so glad you're here," Teri said, smiling at me. I thought she was pretty, but given why we were here, I was pretty sure she didn't think that she was.

"Lisa and Kim are alright," she said, referencing our other two housemates. "But they're kind of attached at the hip and three's a crowd—if you know what I mean."

I hadn't met either Kim or Lisa yet.

"Tonight is menu planning night. You got here just in time."

"Menu planning night?" That sounded interesting. The last time I was here, residents had no say in what was for dinner.

"Yep. We cook our own meals here. We have to do our own grocery shopping, too. Usually two of us cooperate each night to fix the meal. It's a little complicated, trying to fix things that fit easily into everyone's exchanges."

"So we still use exchanges?" That relieved me; I needed something familiar.

"Yes. I'm sure you'll meet with Shannon, the dietician, tomorrow and figure out all your stats. Until then, you'll be happy with what we're having tonight, it's not too bad."

"What is it?" I was curious.

Grinning, Teri chirped, "Veggie burgers, cauliflower with butter, brown rice and sliced peaches. It's my night."

I thought, *a safe dinner, a new friend and relative freedom, maybe this wouldn't be too bad.*

Twenty

Level "3"

I just met with Shannon, my dietician, and I'm in tears. Lord, everything is so much the same. Wait, wait, wait.

"Next Monday we'll see if you've gained weight. You can meet with me again that afternoon," the dietician said.

I couldn't see my weight today either, only on Wednesdays.

Dear God, I know my weight is low, but I'm so scared to gain, and if I have to, can't I have all the details anyway? Please?

No, I want to learn patience and self-control. Please, especially for the next two months, help me to trust you and allow things to vary and be monitored until we know the facts so that I can stay well when I go home. God, help me as I do what I need to do to keep following the rules.

God, even if I lose everyone in the world, I know you will never leave me. You want what's best for me and you will only allow that to happen. I can trust you with my food and activity and my whole life.

* * *

I'd soon learn that a lot of things about my second trip to Remuda were echoes of the first experience.

Like an expert, I catapulted to Level 3 where I was allowed more freedom and given more responsibility. At level one, everything a patient did was monitored and met with skepticism. You weren't even allowed to flush the toilet without a nurse checking to verify that you hadn't purged. But at level three you could even leave The Ranch in groups of two or more.

Half of me wanted to take on the challenges that Level 3 offered, like getting a job in the community or attending civic events. However, I wasn't so thrilled about the requisite restaurant dinners once a week. I remain scarred by one experience.

* * *

I was a little more than halfway through this 60-day stint at Remuda. I'd fallen into routine, even gained a few pounds without freaking out. In fact, just the week before the nurse had finally let me see the number on the scale—a privilege only bestowed upon level 3 patients who were in advanced recovery.

"Abby, I'm so excited we're both on Level 3 now!" Teri bounded into our room where I stood searching my closet, trying to decide what to wear. "I wouldn't worry about getting too dressed up," she said, tossing me a green tank top. "What nice place is going to have space to seat eight women who are weird about food?"

"You're right," I said, slipping the tank over my sun-bleached hair. "I like this shirt because it doesn't make me feel like my stomach sticks out."

"I wouldn't let Julie hear you say that," Teri warned. "She won't let you go on pass tonight. In fact, she'll probably make you sit down and process it all right now."

Julie was therapist to both Teri and me. I loved her. She sported a Tinker Bell hair style. I wished she could just sprinkle some pixie dust on me and make this whole eating disorder go away.

Julie's office, just like Keri's had been, was decked in perky pinks, greens and yellows. I decided it must be some counselors' code to decorate in happy colors. I've never seen an office with red shag carpet or a black leather sofa.

Teri winked, grabbed my hand and tugged me up the hill toward the van.

Shani and Julie were the chaperones for the evening. Chaperones—because even as adult women we couldn't be trusted to clean our plates. We might eat our vegetables, but nothing else. And we weren't beyond throwing a fit over too much salad dressing.

Shani and Julie were along to enforce Remuda's number one rule for challenge events: Everyone must eat all of her sides and at least half of her entrée, no matter what she ordered. We were on a challenge; we weren't supposed to be ordering dinner salads with fat-free dressing.

Shani held the door for the line of girls. We had grown graveyard quiet, each mentally waging war against our personal demons.

"I love the restaurant, Charleston's," Shani told Julie. "My dad used to bring me here on special date nights when I was little. Now I make my boyfriend bring me."

Charleston's didn't usually take reservations, but they made an exception for us. I'm pleased the restaurant was forewarned of our coming, and to put us in the very back corner in case one of us ends up in hysterical tears—and I came close.

Our group sat at a long wooden table; menus open before us.

I looked it over and then whispered in Julie's ear, "There is nothing here I like."

"Find something."

"But seriously, nothing even sounds good."

"Abby, that's part of the challenge. Try something new, or something you didn't like before. You need to get out of your comfort zone. Besides, I think that's probably your eating disorder talking."

No mercy. Could I survive the catastrophic situation I found my in?

The waiter jiggled his pitcher releasing three cubes of ice into my glass. "What can I get for you?"

"Sauerkraut," I replied. I'd never had the stuff, but I knew it was cabbage. Maybe the Rueben sandwich was stuffed full of just cabbage. I could deal with that.

"It comes with coleslaw. Is that okay?"

"Sure," I told him.

"Good job," Julie said. "I'm proud of you."

Thirty minutes later, I had finally melted into casual conversation with the group. Then, the waiter returned guiding another server who could barely see around the huge tray of food he carried. He unceremoniously set my plate in front of me.

I looked down at this thing called dinner. Shreds of cabbage swam in mayonnaise. Agony constricted my stomach, assuring I would not get any of this down. Or, this might be the first time everything came back up.

I sliced my sandwich in unequal halves and deftly picked up the smaller piece.

"I saw that," Julie said sharply.

I ignored Julie and angrily sunk my teeth into the Rueben. Warm layers of beef, spicy sauerkraut and special sauce filled my mouth. Conversation died.

I looked across the table at Teri. She'd gone all out with chicken fried steak. I envied her courage. She was leaving in four days, and I knew she wanted to tackle every possible hurdle while still above Remuda's safety net.

I was leaving in a month. There was still time to avoid the fight.

The evening only got worse. After dinner, Shani pulled the van into the parking lot of an ice cream parlor.

Third in line, I twisted a plastic straw, taken from the restaurant, while I waited my turn. When I reached the counter, I tried to order frozen yogurt, but Julie shot me a "no you don't" look.

"Actually, I don't have enough money for dessert," I lied. "I'll just wait in the van."

"Nope," Julie put her arm around my shoulders and side squeezed: "My treat this time."

* * *

The next morning was a Wednesday, the day I was allowed to glimpse the scale slider as it determined my personal worth.

"Scale, scale, device from hell, tell me what I'm worth."

I lived through that night. In fact, the scale defied all logic and confirmed that I'd lost a quarter pound. How could that be? Relief and horror collided in my chest. I was playing a game with no rules.

Moving to the cul-de-sac didn't change my daily routine, only provided a little distance between the nurses' constant supervision and me. I still had to see my personal therapist, attend group therapy classes and meet with the dietician. My time there was included in the total expected sixty-day stay. Toward the end of those two months, my treatment team, composed of medical doctors and my therapist, would determine if I was healthy enough to go home.

Living with three other adult women accelerated my desire to be out from under parental supervision, to be completely independent and responsible for myself. *I was an adult now! I wanted to be treated as one.*

Two weeks before the end of my sixty days, I began to dread going home to live beneath my parents' roof. In phone conversations they said how excited they were for me to come home and how much they missed me. But I felt it was time to grow up and take care of myself. How could I tell them that I wasn't coming home?

For better or worse, my trip to Remuda Ranch this time around was my emancipation.

"Mom, I'm not moving home." I held the receiver with both sweaty palms.

"What do you mean?" Mom's voice was tinged with uncertainty and fatigue.

"I'm not moving back home when I am discharged."

The pause was long and I feared she had hung up.

Behind me, I could hear Teri and Lisa in the kitchen. Taco salad for dinner, but Teri wanted to stir cheese in with the meat instead of letting each person add their own amount of cheese. I agreed with Lisa, but wasn't in a position to argue at the moment. I sucked in a long breath, noticing that I actually liked the aroma of browning beef.

"Well, there are a couple of things I need to tell you," I said to Mom.

"Should I get your dad on the extension?" Mom asked.

"No, please. Can I just talk to you this time?" Then I told her, "I'm taking my GED tomorrow, for one thing. I'm not going back to high school. In order to continue recovery, when I get home, I'm not going to do anything like what I've been doing in the past."

"What does that mean?" Mom asked.

"It means that I am going to take control of my own life and starting living like an adult. I need you to help me find an apartment so I can move straight into it when I'm discharged."

"Are you kidding?" Mom asked. "Why won't you come home?"

"Mom, I know that my being sick is no one's fault. But the home environment has obviously contributed to me developing and continuing in anorexia. I need a complete change."

"One more thing," I took a deep breath and continued, "I need to get it all out now. I can't go to Israel with you."

Before I had returned to Remuda, my parents had planned a graduation gift for me. Mom and I were scheduled to tour the Holy Lands with Precept Ministries. Both of us had dreamed of this trip for years, and now it loomed an imminent, paid-for reality and I was backing out.

"Mom, as disappointed as I'm sure you are, I don't think I can eat there. It's just not a good time in my recovery for me to take big risks."

"But I thought that was why you were there at Remuda," she said. "You're supposed to learn to eat and live normally again. Is this doing any good? Did you know that your grandparents have paid for this second stint at Remuda? Abby, it's not cheap. If it's not working then why are we doing this?"

Feelings of guilt filled me. As usual, I was failing my family, crushing everyone's expectations of me.

Once again, I became compliant—which I knew to be a dangerous sign. I renewed my ploy to "I play by the rules," only to fulfill every requirement of treatment, but vowed that my loyalty would be to the call of my anorexia. And I could hear it calling me once again. Its voice was louder than was my desire to please my parents or even the treatment team.

I would wait until I was discharged to do things my own way again. I was an adult. I could and would do things my way.

This time, relapse promised to be even easier.

* * *

Yesterday we celebrated my birthday and as always, I cried—again— because of my eating disorder. Mom and Dad are so worried, but God, I'm not willing to change. What's wrong with me?

I feel really ugly, nasty, and worthless. I didn't deserve birthday gifts or a celebration, but people gave me stuff anyway.

Oh God, I can't stand it. I'm going to kill myself. I want to be well for my family. I want to eat normally for them. I want my life to blend in with everyone else's, so that I won't be such a problem anymore. For as long as I can remember, I've been contrary—at odds with the normal people. If being well is so "right" and "good" and what everyone who loves me wants, how come I don't want it?

I don't want to change, or to be healthy. Why don't I even want to weigh a healthy, energetic, comfortable weight?

How long until my folks give up and abandon me?

Twenty-One

The Letter

A lot of things changed while I was at Remuda. This time, my family moved to Wichita, Kansas, because Dad took a full-time position with one of his consulting clients.

I was accepted to Oklahoma State University with my GED and ACT score, so I got my wish and moved out of my parents' house mere months after I returned from The Ranch.

Much as I craved it, complete independence did not prove to be good for me. No one held me accountable to my meal plan. No one was there to chastise me for going running at five in the morning. Almost immediately, I reverted to my anorexic habits like a security blanket. It was all I really knew to do. I identified myself as anorexic. Left alone what else could I do, but whittle down my meals and go for another run?

My sister Jennifer recalls how thin I'd become a mere five months later. "After we moved to Wichita, that was the scariest time. You looked like a walking skeleton and people in Stillwater kept calling Mom and Dad. They would see you out running and be concerned. I even remember a story of you not thinking you could afford to buy cold medicine and I was upset because you acted like Mom and Dad didn't care for us or take care of us. You would fall asleep almost every time you sat down and the only indication of you waking up was the resuming of your leg bouncing. I dreamed I was at your funeral and I was really afraid you would die soon."

* * *

A lesser love would have given up on me long ago, but I was blessed to be surrounded with family fueled by the unconditional love of Christ.

My maternal grandparents were central to my growing-up years. Before I got sick, my sisters and I spent hours in the workshop with

Granddad or playing cards and dominoes in their sunroom. Of course we never visited them without Granddad making his famous chocolate malt, or sharing one of his dark chocolate Dove ice cream bars.

Granddad loved food and was enormously frustrated by my refusal to eat. He also lived life passionately and couldn't understand why I didn't see the connection between food and life, starving and dying.

In October, five months after I left the Arizona residential treatment center, Granddad wrote me a letter, desperate to convince me that life was worth living. I don't remember receiving the letter. Fifteen years later, it fell from the folds of my journal.

Dear Abby,

I've started a dozen or more "almost letters" to you recently and there may be that many more (with them all being "almost sent," too) before one that seems acceptable results. All have had the same objective and all wanting the best for you. All not wanting to sound offensive. All wanting to help, but all written with a sense of helplessness and fear of being received other than as intended. This is but another effort. Please be patient with its author.

Pages could be filled with well-deserved plaudits of every kind for you, your personal life, your accomplishments and your potential. While passed over here for brevity sake, be aware, they are recognized and all around you as they have been for many, many years.

This note, however is simply one of concern—almost completely of concern. Concern that you may have your priorities out of order. Concern that you appear to almost be testing God. Neither is desirable. Neither effective. Both affecting you, your future and your very life and the lives of your family and friends. Before you throw this aside wondering "what next?" would you feel it out of line to try as best you could to help a loved one who was chaining his or herself to a pillar in a building set for demolition. If so, chuck it, but give me a chance.

Abby you were given a healthy body capable of almost all human desires and needs and, thankfully, of enduring substantial abuse as well. God only asks that you care for it and use it to His glory. You did for many years. For some reason, whether by outside influences or factors of unknown source or power, its care became a "forgotten" aspect of your life and its ability to withstand abuse significantly tested. Some of its important capabilities may have already been sacrificed.

You know God loves you and wants nothing but the best for you and that He is always ready to help. His help usually is accomplished by His acting through others, e.g., doctors, family, friends or even strangers or the most unlikely. And, while spectacular miracles still happen, more often His help is accomplished in less flamboyant fashions (His love for us and help, however given, being miraculous in itself). This is the area in which you seem in some ways to be testing God or waiting for Him to "do it all." Hopefully, I'm wrong and in any case I'm sure it's not being done consciously, but, if this, consciously or unconsciously, is preventing your use of your knowledge of what is necessary, or from using advice and accepting help from those you know are right and ready to help, then the other concern comes to the surface: the concern of priorities.

Nothing other than your love of God at this point is more important than your health and that requires a solid, balanced, diet, plenty of rest and reasonable exercise, all geared to your state of and obtained well-being. Now! Not after or along with work, not after or along with school, not after or along with anything that prevents or detracts from the regiment required for you to regain your health. If you need someone to hold you still, keep you in bed, watch you constantly for diversions or detractions, or fix acceptable food —24 hours a day if needed and until you regain a reasonable sate of health and ability to maintain it by yourself. You need only ask and mean it. (At your age today, Abby, you would have to ask and accept such guardianship or overseeing unless things are allowed to reach the state of requiring some court to accomplish such consent.) You can have most anything "out there" but not in your present state of health and anything that would be necessary to be "put off" in order for you to regain your health will only be that much better with you healthy.

Your faith is capable as is your God,

Love, The ends G of G & G with 1st G's concurrence

I was 33 when I found that letter. I probably opened it the first time standing alone in my fourth floor dorm room at Oklahoma State University. Then tucked it in my journal frustrated at another demand that I "just eat!" With a malnourished mind, I completely forgot about the letter.

Twenty-Two

A College Student at Last!

How I loved my grandfather. He was wise and kind and wanted the best for me. Like my parents, he hoped and expected that I'd attend college. He was pleased that I chose Oklahoma State University, the same place that my mother, her two brothers and even my father had attended.

I wish I could say that in starting college all of my priorities came together. I wish I could say that I became so involved in challenging classes and the social nature of campus that I forgot about achieving abstract, bodily perfection. I know this happens with some people; it didn't for me.

Going to college was nonnegotiable in my family. While they didn't have a preference as to where we went, from the time we were little, my parents had made it clear to my sisters and me that we were expected to go to college.

I completed my senior year at Stillwater High School, even though I had technically already "graduated" with my GED. Since I wasn't allowed to walk across the stage with my peers at the formal graduation ceremony, my parents held a small party for me at home.

I went through college on some days feeling like two people and on others, feeling like half a person. The soul of me floated above, helpless and inert, watching my flesh make foolish choices and sink deeper into despair.

My soul screamed and wondered at my body's deafness. She pleaded, "Why won't you just stop? Just eat? Just be normal?"

At Oklahoma State, freshmen students are required to live either in the dorms or with their parents. Getting my own apartment was not an option, and since my family had just moved to Kansas I had no choice. But to move into a college dorm, I submitted my application for housing at the last minute and was assigned to the fourth floor of Bennet

Hall. Every night I felt like Cinderella, climbing the clock tower to her lonely abode. Of course, I never took the elevator.

For the first two weeks, I had a roommate, but she rather quickly moved into another dorm across campus. Shannon's move left me with the accommodations every anorexic dreams of: solitude, no supervision and a built-in workout from the bottom floor to my live-in closet multiple times per day.

Now alone, I happily got on with my solitary life. My parents had purchased the mandatory meal card so that I could eat in the Student Union, and though I had classmates who frequently invited me to join them, I always preferred dining alone.

The fourth floor of Bennett was sparsely populated, but the other girls stayed up late watching movies, started an intramural soccer league and snuck scented candles past the Resident Administrator.

Keeping to myself as much as I could, I didn't make many friends.

My days pretty much followed the same routine: I woke at 5:30 every morning that first semester in order to fit in a run around Boomer Lake before my 7:30 Spanish class. Each morning, I fought to stay awake in all three morning classes, and then I'd hop on my bike and pedal to my job at the Red Lobster, to work the lunch shift. After busing my last table, I'd rush back to campus for my class on journalistic reporting.

I rarely studied. The act of sitting and staring at a text book practically demands snack food and I never allowed myself to eat anything before 7 p.m. What if by the end of the day I overate? No, best to simply wait until the last minute when I could fall in bed after eating and not risk losing control.

Every single night after my shift at Red Lobster, I piled a Styrofoam box with iceberg lettuce and twelve sliced Roma tomatoes. I doused my salad with red wine vinegar and grabbed 200 calories of Saltine crackers. I stood by my dresser to eat, listening to the radio. Finally I collapsed in bed with a bulging belly, burning with the acid from diet Pepsi, vinegar, tomatoes and salt.

With a full class load, I held down two jobs. I needed to not need Daddy's help paying for school. I wanted my parents to see that I could be self-sufficient.

Twenty-Three

House Hunting

I lived in Bennett Hall my entire freshman year. The sweaty halls of its sparsely populated fourth floor and the lonely hallways fit my mood.

In my mind, the harder and the more difficult something was, the better I liked it. Just like restricting my food intake, I practiced asceticism in all aspects of life. I didn't need comfort. I believed that enduring the oppressive heat barely alleviated by my wimpy window fan made me a stronger person. Isolation, self-imposed relational restriction, made me a better person than those who leaned on each other.

However, by summer break that year, loneliness set in.

One afternoon I bumped into a high school friend in the Student Center's coffee shop who offered an alternative.

"Oh my gosh, Abby, I haven't seen you in ages! I wasn't even sure you stayed in Stillwater for college. How are you?" Nellie wasn't normally a gushy person and I knew from experience that she hated hugs. All the same she seemed genuinely happy to see me.

"I'm fine, just busy. How are you?" I accepted my black, half-decaf Americano and turned to face her. "Want anything? My treat."

"No, I'm good. But hey, running into you gives me an idea. I lived with my folks for my freshman year, but I'm ready to get out. Working with them at their appliance store, and living with them is too much." She shrugged a bulging backpack higher on her shoulders and we headed toward the computer lab.

"I love your folks," I interjected. Her mom was the craziest dog-lady I'd ever met, except for maybe Nellie herself. They threw annual birthday parties for their Shih Tzu, inviting guests, baking special cakes from scratch and perching pink party hats on the furry heads.

"Yeah, they're great in small doses." She smiled. "So I'm looking for a place, but I really need a roommate to afford it. Where are you living? Would you be interested in renting a small house with me?"

I flashed back to a recent conversation with my mom.

"Abby, the resident assistant from your dorm called. I think she said her name is Robin."

"So?"

"A few of the girls on your floor came to her and expressed concern for you."

"Why? I'm fine! Besides, I'm hardly ever there!"

"She said they're worried because you're so thin. They think you might be throwing up in the bathroom, too. Have you started purging?"

"Absolutely not!" I was furious, and felt betrayed by my floor mates who didn't even know me. And I especially felt betrayed by Robin, who brought this up to my parents without talking to me. And I was hurt that my mom would question me like this.

"They aren't taking any action right now, but I think Robin was suggesting you find another place to live. Your precarious health is making the other girls uncomfortable."

I reached ahead of Nellie to open the heavy computer lab door. Knowing her preference to keep to herself meant that she wouldn't harass me about my habits, my weight or failing efforts at recovery.

"Sharing a house with you—I'd love to," I told her. "Do you want to house hunt this weekend?"

That night I wrote in my journal, *Are you out to get me, God? Life stinks! One more decision or demand and I'm going to crash and burn. All I want is to go to bed. Can't you just kill me?*

Twenty-Four

Homeward Bound—Again

Thankfully, and wondrously, I managed to keep good grades in college. I graduated in the four years with a degree in public relations, but honestly, the classes are a hazy memory at best. My malnourished body could barely keep my heart beating, let alone aid my brain in handling the rigors of academia.

Routine is what saved me—operating within a groove of carefully guarded habits. Methodically, day after day, after a demanding morning workout, I walked to class where the instant my butt hit the seat I would nod off. I often wonder what my teachers thought about that.

Nellie and I had found a house on Husband Street. It was in better shape than some other rentals we looked at nearby, but it also left much to be desired. But affordability ruled the day. When we talked Cassie—who was in the journalism program with me—into being a third roommate, the house was easily affordable.

I liked the house because it was a good four blocks from the very edge of campus. Coming home between classes as often as I could, added to my daily mileage and subsequent calorie burn. Red Lobster, where I still waited tables, was a little farther, but no more than a 10-minute bike ride.

Nellie and I decided to take a class together. We picked astronomy, something fun and unrelated to either of our majors.

"It's at 4 p.m. on Tuesdays and Thursdays," Nellie said.

"I can do that," I said, glancing at the catalogue she referenced, bouncing on my toes as we stood there together—because I never miss an opportunity to burn an extra calorie. "It's only a 45 minute class, right? I like to work the dinner shift at Red Lobster whenever I can, so it looks like the class would be over in time for me to get to my job at the restaurant."

"It has a lab too, but it's only homework, no specific time, so we can work it in. I'm going on-line and registering for it now."

"I'll do it tomorrow," I told her. "I'm headed to Boomer Lake for an afternoon walk."

Nellie didn't look up. "You're crazy," she said. "You never sit still."

* * *

By now, I was a sophomore. Nellie and I walked to class together the first Tuesday afternoon of that year. Astronomy was really interesting, or at least what I remember of it. Although Nellie would laugh about my sleeping in class, she didn't want me as a study partner from then on. In fact, she turned me down as a lab partner. "I'm sorry, Abby, but you sleep through class every week. I don't know how you're making an A. I can't worry about your work affecting my grade."

Nonetheless, I finished the class with an A—but my friendship with Nellie had grown chilly.

Cassie turned out to be an awful roommate. By the end of the semester, Nellie and I were at our wits end putting up with her dogs and boyfriend. Fortuitously, Nellie's sister was moving, so we jumped at the chance to rent her house on the outskirts of town. There was no way I could walk to class now, but the lightly trafficked roads were perfect for long runs.

Nellie's cousin, Marc, transferred to Oklahoma State University the next semester and she invited him to live with us. Marc was nice enough, but I didn't know him and felt uncomfortable being at the house with him when she was gone. So I moved into my own apartment at the end of my sophomore year.

Now living in Wichita, my parents continued to fret, because their friends called and gave them updates about my weight. "I saw Abby out running at Boomer. She doesn't look good."

And so Mom called. "Abby, we keep hearing stories that you're not doing well at all."

"I'm fine, Mom," I insisted. "Who's spying on me anyway?"

"No one is spying on you and it doesn't matter who told me. Your dad and I have made up our minds. Either you put school on hold in order to go inpatient again, or you rearrange your schedule so that you can come see the counselor of our choice here in Wichita."

"Fine," I whimpered into the phone. "I'll talk to my advisor about taking only Tuesday and Thursday classes next semester. Do you think I can see the therapist on Friday afternoons?"

"Probably, but Abby, I want you to stay here over the weekend, too."

"Mom, I need to come back to Stillwater so I can work."

"You do not have to work." Mom said. "We don't trust you right now to eat. At least if you're here through the weekend, I can help hold you accountable. Don't you know how much we love you? Your dad and I are so afraid right now."

In spite of my outward resistance, something in me was grateful for Mom's words. I guess I was at least willing to admit to myself that I was drowning under the burden of a heavy class load and thirty to forty hours per week at the restaurant, what social life I did have—and, the never-ending work of tending to my anorexia.

Surprised that I so easily and willingly would place myself back under the scrutiny of my family, made me aware that I had unilaterally made a decision to once again make a concerted effort to regain my health. But I knew that being at home with my family would lighten my burden, and give me the anchor I needed to beat the predatory lies of anorexia.

Twenty-Five

Rachelle's Sweet Gift

Filled with conflict and anxiety, nonetheless, each Thursday evening, I made the exactly two-hour drive to my family's home in Wichita.

Resilient, my parents managed to reestablish a modicum of peace and continuity between my visits.

Family life when I was away at college had naturally found a rhythm based around a growing family. My sisters were busy with normal kid things. Rachelle excelled in gymnastics and Kelsey found her niche in soccer. Jenny flourished academically and athletically. It was possible to plan on the spur of the moment—such as heading out to Sonic for cherry limeades. No one cried over breakfast.

But then, enter Abby! When I arrived, it was as if someone laid a carpet of eggshells. Everyone tiptoed around me, never sure what to say, never sure when I might burst into tears. I was on edge, protective of all the habits I so carefully practiced in Stillwater when I had no supervision. Now my parents confronted me about my early morning workouts and personalized dinners. When I was home, my sisters struggled to live normally on the periphery of a raging storm, while I once again commanded the bulk of my parents' attention.

One Friday afternoon Mom asked me to pick up Rachelle from Folger's gym where she had gymnastics practice.

"Chelle finishes at four, so you can easily swing by and pick her up on your way home from counseling with Tamara," mom had said.

Tamara. I really liked her. She was associated with the PATH Clinic in Wichita. My mother had found her in the yellow pages, one of the only Christian therapists specializing in eating disorders in the area. Tamara was simple in every way. Her office was cool and dark, windowless in the back of an office complex. She didn't ordain her walls with large posters of daisies and Bible verses like Keri and Julynn. No hot-pink *Koosh* ball to worry my fingers through.

It was under her leadership that I saw a new development within me. Recovery, I realized, was something I had to do for myself. Slowly, but surely, I began to take ownership of, and responsibility for my eating disorder. As this new-found discovery was evolving, my wearied parents began to ease up on their ever-present vigilance of me.

And an empathy for them set in. Up to this point, I had fought them tooth and nail. Poor parents; I had caused them never-ending worry.

But here I was, responsible enough to be told to go pick up my sister. I drove along, with the heater going full blast. It was sweltering outside, and yet I was chilled to the bone. Even the rays of the long summer sun failed to warm me. Folding my bony body into the driver's seat of Dad's Bonneville, the heater at full blast, I placed each hand alternately in front of the heater to warm myself. Ten minutes later I pulled into the parking lot of Rachelle's gym.

"Hi, Abby! I didn't know you were picking me up."

"Hey, Sunshine!" I had given her that nickname when she was barely two. The name fit her, irrepressibly bubbly, full of life. "Yep, best part of my day."

She tossed her bulky gym bag in the trunk, opened the passenger door and swung herself into my hotbox.

"Abby, it's so hot in here! How can you breathe?"

"I'm not hot. Tamara's office was so cold I'll probably never thaw out."

Rachelle surveyed my attire. Blue jeans, a long sleeved t-shirt and an Oklahoma State hoodie. She punched the button on the dash changing the clock to reflect the outdoor temperature: 103.

I was nearly twenty years old, approaching six years of hardcore battle with anorexia.

Rachelle was only ten. Years later she confessed to me that in the car that afternoon—seeing me chilled to the bone while surrounded by 103 degrees of heat—was the first time the gravity of my situation fully dawned on her.

Precious Rachelle. Because of her innocence, and our age difference, Rachelle's gift to me was like no other. She never looked at me with sad, questioning eyes. She never begged me to eat. She never refused to go for a walk with me, afraid I'd burn too many calories. Rachelle looked at me with untainted affection.

My parents weren't in a position to love me without concern for my life. Their God-ordained role was to protect me and teach me to be a self-sufficient adult. But Rachelle played an equally important role in my recovery. She helped me to retain my dignity—and eventually to reclaim my role as her "big sister."

Twenty-Six

"One Day"

One of the most precious memories of my college days happened every Tuesday night. A hodge-podge gathering of students met in the sanctuary of University Heights Baptist Church for student-led praise and worship. I became an unofficial member of their small group. In the early summer between my sophomore and junior year of college the church's college group planned to attend a Christian conference called *One Day*.

One Day was held on a rural farm in Tennessee. College students from around the country gathered for a single night of camping under the stars, for a unique worship experience and to listen to renowned Christian speakers such as Chris Tomlin and Louie Giglio.

I fought the college pastor tooth and nail. "I don't have time to go to this *One Day* conference in Tennessee. I need to work; I need to study."

Tina gave me a skeptical look. She wouldn't understand if I admitted that I was afraid of the bus ride, fast food restaurants and camping. Where would I do my morning workout? Did she have any idea how many calories are in a Big Mac?

However, three days later I found myself in a church van with twelve other hyper college students, driving from Oklahoma to Tennessee for *One Day*.

Most of that trip is a blur in my mind. I remember very little except for one song, the one night we camped at Shelby Farms-and one mysterious woman.

We arrived at Shelby Farms shortly before sunset and rushed to set up our tents. As soon as our little plot of land was secured, we followed the crowd of other students converging on a hillside facing a makeshift stage. There, Chris Tomlin had begun to strum his guitar softly, welcoming the crowd into an attitude of worship.

The organizers of the conference had arranged to call Botswana, Africa, and share our worship with them. As the students on this side of the ocean began to sing, "We Fall Down," Christians on the other side of the world joined the chorus in their own language.

I hung back, not feeling particularly conversational or even happy to be there. I found a fallen tree and lay down on my stomach to cry and to pray.

My heart wrenched with sorrow, exhaustion and hopelessness. I pleaded with God. "God there's nothing else I can do. There's nothing else that counselors can tell me or doctors can suggest. I'm dying and I can't stop. God, God, please do something."

I have no idea what she looked like, and I can't remember her voice, but a woman came up behind me and wrapped her arms around me. She allowed me to pour out my despair. I don't remember if she counseled or encouraged me, or if she simply listened.

When we parted and I returned to the tent that evening, something felt different. I identified the unfamiliar pangs of hunger. I didn't try to explain it to anyone, but sat by the campfire marveling at a mystery that had taken place inside of me. I pulled an unwound coat hanger from the flames and reached for a hotdog.

I attribute this incident, as much as any other, as a milestone for me. *One Day* marked the close of anorexia's predatory hold over me. On this day, I stepped into the light of recovering. On this day, I did believe that I could recover from the life-threatening jaws of anorexia.

I could climb out of the mire of self-starvation, loneliness and hopelessness.

My life could have a happy ending.

Back in Stillwater, a mere 72 hours later, I didn't look any different. I hadn't gained an ounce and I still went for my morning run. But God had broken the chains of my disease, and I began to understand that nothing I could ever do or achieve would make me self-sufficient.

Twenty-Seven

The Marriage Proposal

I walked in the light of the all sufficiency of Jesus for the next five years.

But my old long-standing predatory friend—Anorexia Nervosa—was not yet willing to give me up. In the form of pride, he came after saying, "You can do this on your own; you don't need anyone."

At first I bought into it.

If I was going to give up anorexia, it had to be on my terms. It could not look as if I failed as an anorexic, or as if someone took it from me. It could not appear as if I'd grown weak, lost my resolve or no longer had the self-discipline to push my body beyond healthy limits. If I was going to recover, it was going to be according to my plan, my way and my timing.

But the experience of *One Day* had been powerful. Maybe, just maybe, God could remove the chains of anorexia from me. And keep His everlasting promise, *"Therefore, if anyone is in Christ, he is a new creation. The old has passed away; behold, the new has come"* (2 Corinthians 5:17).

God would remind of this from time to time, such as years later, when He would have me revisit the moment of my truth as a reminder that it is through Him and from Him that all blessings flow.

In the car one afternoon, I randomly popped a CD into the CD player. Tracks melted into the air, slipping past my consciousness until track 10. In the live recording, Chris Tomlin announced, "We are going to call Botswana, Africa, and you're going to hear them singing "We Fall Down" with us, in their own language." It was the recording of that very same day I had stood tearfully on a hill at Shelby Farms. With that song, God strengthened my heart and reminded me that He had not forgotten me and was intentionally involved in my moments.

My eternal Heavenly Father played the melody that recalled for me the day He broke the chains that bound me to anorexia.

It wouldn't be the last of God's gifts to me.

He would send me love in the form a husband.

And then I met someone who would become my husband. Ironically, I met him in a kitchen. Not one where I ate, but in the back of Red Lobster, where he was a cook and I was a waitress. Patrick and I both attended Stillwater High School, and then found ourselves at Oklahoma State University, and working part-time at the restaurant.

It happened right after my epiphany at *One Day* in Tennessee. I was doing pretty well, maintaining a healthy weight, and beginning to feel sexy and confident.

One late November afternoon, the restaurant staff stood hovering over the schedule for Thanksgiving weekend. Patrick and I had the holiday off and didn't have to work again until the big football game on Saturday night. Everyone worked game nights.

"You should come home with me for Thanksgiving." The words fell out of my mouth before they even crossed my mind. I almost choked when I heard myself. "It's always at my grandparents' house in Bartlesville so it would mean staying overnight."

To that point, we'd never been on a date, in fact, we'd scarcely interacted except for a few coy winks between the warming lamps and the food prep station at Red Lobster.

"That sounds fun," he answered. "My family doesn't really do much for Thanksgiving." That was not the truth I would later learn, but it confirmed that he really was interested in spending time with me.

My grandparents' house was stuffed to the gills with extended family. Patrick found himself surrounded by my cousins and grilled by my dad and grandfather. He was in the National Guard and the ROTC program at OSU, preparing to commission as an infantry officer. My non-military family was fascinated by his ambition.

Patrick was quiet, reserved, and stoic, so by the time we drove back to Stillwater on Friday night, I was certain I would never hear from him again.

But I did.

Patrick had not only survived the holiday, but was intrigued enough to call again.

I knew immediately that he was the man I would marry.

On some level, Patrick knew I had a problem. Though scarcely acquaintances, we had met one another in high school. He'd seen me rail thin like everyone else, and had noticed that I disappeared for three months during my senior year. But it never registered that all this might be due to anorexia, a diagnosable mental illness.

Two years would pass, and then, during a Thanksgiving break two years after our first memorable "date," Patrick asked me to marry him.

I said, "Yes!"

Since I was a year behind him in school, he graduated, commissioned and left for his first duty station, Fort Bragg, North Carolina. I remained in Stillwater to finish my college classes.

And began to plan our wedding.

I was fairly relaxed in planning the wedding, and not particularly concerned with the "perfect wedding." I mean, I certainly couldn't care less about the cake; I wasn't going to eat any.

Even before the wedding, our relationship endured a lot. Deployment to Iraq loomed close on Patrick's horizon, so the 82nd Airborne forbid him to return to Kansas where our wedding plans were in their final stages.

He called me one afternoon with the bad news. "I can't come home for the wedding."

"What do you mean you can't come home? It's your wedding!" I was in the car with one of my best friends, the window down, passing by a frozen yogurt store and she wanted to stop. I waved her to keep going.

"My unit is preparing to deploy," he explained. "I'm not allowed to be more than two hours away from Fort Bragg."

"I'll call you back this evening," Patrick was still talking. "It will be okay, I promise. Let me ask around about a few things, but I have an idea."

By December, six months later, we had moved the wedding to the east coast and arranged for the Army chaplain to perform the ceremony on the military Base. The chapel came pre-decorated, full of Christmas ribbon, holly and candles.

Our rehearsal dinner was at Ci-Ci's pizza and our honeymoon was on the floor of our new, unfurnished house. Patrick scavenged the construction sites in our fledgling neighborhood for scraps of wood and built a fire. That first night we snuggled into sleeping bags with full glasses of real, full-fat eggnog.

Our wedding album testifies to a brief hiatus from anorexia's ravages on my body. I felt so beautiful that day; why couldn't I internalize the truth that I was beautiful at a healthy weight?

Why was my recovery so fragile?

Two months later, on Valentine's Day, Patrick left for a year in Iraq. I stayed alone, setting up house in the tiny town of Raeford, North Carolina.

I wanted to be in control. I wanted everyone to see that I had my life, health, marriage and future under control.

My disease was still talking to me—once again trying to convince me I didn't need any help.

Twenty-Eight

Promises, Promises

After our wedding, I maintained a healthy weight for three years. However, in my heart I still bowed to a culture that demanded pride in my appearance. I continued to work out to prove, if only to myself, my superior self-discipline, physical strength and will power.

While I loved my husband and was excited about our new life, I was still preoccupied with my idea of a perfect self—which still included a strict adherence to my weight. In other words, the "anorexia thinking" remained.

In August of 2005, while Patrick was in Afghanistan, my mom invited me to join her at Precept Ministry's annual Bible conference in Chattanooga, Tennessee. There messages by Ravi Zacharias, Janet Parshal, Max Lucado, Kay Arthur and others, struck home. They spoke about resisting idolatry, of Nehemiah standing armed and resilient against all foes, committed to restoring the city of Jerusalem and her surrounding wall. The message spoke to me, and I understood the point as it related to my preoccupation with the image of my body.

I felt humbled, convicted of my weakness to withstand my own idol and rebuild the health of my body, which according to Scripture is God's temple. The three-day conference concluded at noon on Sunday

"Thanks for attending this with me here," Mom said, giving me a hug as we stood by my car. "Thanks, too, for dropping me off at the airport. It sure beats taking a cab!"

"I'm so, so glad we did this." I hugged her back. It felt good knowing that my weight gain meant she couldn't count my ribs as we embraced.

"Maybe we can make this an annual thing," Mom suggested, lingering through the passenger side window. "It would be fun to look forward to it."

"I'd like that. But I better hit the road. It looks like a monsoon is about to strike and I'd rather not do the last half of my eight hour drive in the rain and the dark."

We each blew a kiss and I drove away.

Finally being a healthy weight made me feel better, and had banished the proverbial elephant from the room—and contributed to much improved relationships. In fact, our relationship was blossoming into genuine friendship.

Still, I knew she and Daddy still worried about me, but the overriding fear of a midnight call informing them that their daughter had died of malnutrition was gone.

For my part, my weight was safely balanced between just heavy enough and not too scary. While I was busy learning to enjoy aspects of married life and was experiencing more satisfaction with life in general, the numbers on the scale had climbed. Marriage, it seemed, and a new home and new friends and all, had eclipsed the nagging voice of anorexia.

Hallelujah to that! Maybe I could beat this after all.

The drive home was far from monotonous. Rain drilled my car so loudly that I couldn't hear the radio or the books on tape that I had brought to pass the time. But it gave me time to think, and the introspection was productive. God was beckoning me to listen to Him about the things I had learned at the conference.

I began to pray out loud.

Then, I began to sing my prayer at the top of my lungs, partially in expression of my sincerity, partially to stay awake and partially because I couldn't hear myself over the rain otherwise.

But God was insistent. His voice rose above the cacophony of raindrops, and up and over the sound of my words. He spoke specifically to my situation. I love that about the Heavenly Father. Nehemiah 7:5 says, "God put it in my heart." That's what He did for me that afternoon. As soon as I got home, I scribbled my commitment to God in my journal:

I will be content with exercising only one day per week;
I will pray and spend time with God every day before I workout;
I will not workout for longer than I spend with God;
I will study and memorize the Bible continually; and,
I will not have any long-range workout programs.

I put the journal on my nightstand, a daily reminder of my promise to God.

On one level, sharing with God the "simple" tasks I promised to uphold seemed silly. Does God really care about the length and location of my workouts? He does, of course. He is my Heavenly Father, and I am His child. He loves me.

In Exodus 20, God commands us to have no other Gods beside Him. For me, banishing my false gods involved quitting the gym, establishing accountability in my food intake and uncompromising limits on my exercise. Everything that factored into my insatiable desire for a perfect body, had to go.

And so I entered into a covenant with God. A covenant is an agreement between two or more persons to do or not do something specified. Throughout the Old Testament, God made covenants with His people. And so He made a covenant with me. If I would obey His specific commands, He would take care of all my needs, including those of my physical body.

I believed this will all my heart. And remained steadfast to the promise.

Steadily, against deeply ingrained fears, I obeyed God's personal commands for my health.

But within two years, just like the Israelites, I was distracted by the glitter of ordinary idols and their false promises. For me, the idols were about stressing out over a combination of fears due to several life changes such as the responsibility of managing the frequent packing up one house and a move to a new state, then setting up yet a new home with the constantly being new to a community and not knowing anyone was all a bit much; this drove me further to seek comfort in the familiar. With anorexic behaviors I felt a sense of personal control—even when my world turned upside down. And so I began to slide back into the grip of anorexia's demands that my full attention to the weight of my body was what mattered most in my life.

It was a terrible spiral. I found myself kneeling again before a heartless idol of physical perfection. Here I was, once again, on the brink of dying from a malnourished body.

I knew that God had rescued me from anorexia once. For a few brief years, I had experienced the freedom that He wanted for me. More than anything, I wanted to worship and honor Him with my mind and body. Why was I still so attracted by this idol of physical "perfection"?

Conflict consumed me, and so I turned to Philippians 3:18-21, for strength. *"For, as I have often told you before and now say again even with tears, many live as enemies of the cross of Christ. Their destiny is destruction, their god is their stomach, and their glory is in their shame. Their mind is on earthly things. But our citizenship is in heaven. And we eagerly await a Savior from there, the Lord Jesus Christ, who, by the power that enables him to bring everything under his control, will transform our lowly bodies so that they will be like his glorious body."*

And to soothe and feed my heart and soul, I turned to Isaiah 30:21-22: *"And your ears shall hear a word behind you saying, 'This is the way, walk in it,' when you turn to the right or when you turn to the left. Then you will defile your idols overlaid with silver and your gold-plated metal images. You will scatter them as unclean things. You will say to them, 'Be gone!'"*

I pleaded with God to make this true in my own life. I wanted to demand that anorexia "be gone!" It seemed ironic that I could possess such will power to resist food and yet be so weak when it came to ending the eating disorder. I needed God to work supernaturally, because I wasn't able to help myself.

Twenty-Nine

A Starving Marriage

Patrick deployed from Fort Bragg twice. First for a year to Iraq, beginning two months after our wedding. The second deployment was to Afghanistan in 2005, less than two years later.

In March 2006, after 3 years, 3 months of marriage, my husband and I moved to Columbus, Georgia, so that he could attend the Captain's Career Course at Fort Benning.

I knew when we got married that soldiers and their families lead transient lives, but I didn't grasp what that really means for daily life, until our move to Georgia. By then I had settled into my church and our neighborhood, my job at General Nutrition Centers and our house in North Carolina.

I was completely unprepared for the terrible loneliness that struck me when we got to Georgia. As soon as the boxes were unpacked and put away in our 940 square foot apartment, I began a frantic search for something more to do other than being a stay-at-home wife.

"Abby, I don't know why you're looking for a job," my husband said one evening as he changed out of his uniform. I was fixing dinner.

"We're going to live here a year if that. Why don't you volunteer somewhere instead? Besides, when we find a church, you'll make friends there."

I didn't answer. A million options were already pinging around in my head. I would set all of them in motion and see which ones came through. By the end of the week I would not be bored. I refused to be idle for one minute; it made me feel worthless and lazy, a dangerously similar feeling to how I felt in the eating disorder.

The following Sunday, I sat at our computer in the office while Patrick studied at the kitchen table less than eight feet away. Still looking for something to occupy time, I was hoping to find a fun 5K to run, thinking that at least I would meet people with whom I would have similar interests.

Google's results weren't exactly what I was looking for, but in my desperation, what it offered seemed even better: The Columbus Road Runners running club. I scanned the webpage: *Various group runs throughout the week. Email Mike for locations, times and alternate routes.*

I shuttled a note through cyberspace to Mike, wondering if I'd hear back anytime soon. Within seconds, he replied. "Great to hear from you. Always happy to have new runners. We meet tomorrow morning at 5:45 for an easy seven miles." He provided directions to the event, and signed off with, "See you tomorrow."

I felt committed, but anxious about running seven miles and starting so early. Who goes running before the sun comes up? But I was challenged. I set the alarm for 4:30 a.m. and placed my Nikes by the front door.

The Columbus Road Runners club ended up being both the best and the worst thing that happened to me the entire two and a half years my husband and I lived in Georgia. Through the running club, I made fast friends and established routine around the scheduled runs. At the same time, the innate competition to be the best, the fastest and go the farthest caused me to lose weight quickly.

That first run, I found myself straggling behind a group of five men somewhere between my dad's age and my own. But they were kind and encouraging.

"You did great for never having run more than six miles before," John told me when we finished. "I think you're the fastest female we've ever had join us."

"Seriously," Mac chimed in, "actually, the real test is next week. Usually the women never show up a second time."

I glowed under their admiration. "I'll be back," I promised.

I was hungry for the assurance of commonality and friendship. The wives of soldiers enrolled in the career course had already been warned that our husbands were going to be virtually unavailable for the entirety of the course. The running club sounded promising.

"There's also a group of girls that meet on Thursdays," Mike offered. "They're slower than us," he winked, "but a pretty good group."

"So, are you going to join us Wednesday?" Reynolds spoke for the first time. He was the tallest one, quiet with an aura of gentle strength. I never learned whether Reynolds was his first or last name.

"What happens Wednesday?" I asked.

"It's our first 14 miler of the year," Mike, always exuberant, answered. "We meet out at Schomburg High School at 6 a.m."

"There's no way I can run 14 miles," I tried to laugh, but instantly felt a sense of failure.

"Sure you can," John encouraged. "Fourteen miles is not that much different than seven miles, especially when the sun is not even up yet, and the time and distance fly by. Besides, you can turn around part way if you want."

Their faith in me buoyed my pride and a desire to accept the challenge. It also helped to squelch the warning in my gut that was saying, "You have no business running 14 miles. You are learning to put exercise in perspective; this is not healthy for you."

I didn't want to listen. The idols of pride, self-sufficiency and a hunger for approval glittered before me. I took small steps toward it, one longer run at a time.

Almost before I knew it, I was running over 20 miles every Saturday and cresting the 50 mile mark every week.

As quickly as my mileage increased, my weight plummeted. I still shunned the scale like therapists had taught me in the treatment programs I had attended. But this time it was because I was afraid that the scale would show the loss of weight so drastic that I'd be sent straight back to the hospital.

So I ignored the truth. Because my husband and I lived hundreds of miles from family, no one was there to call me to account my weight loss, nor the extreme measures of running that was contributing to the weight loss.

Perhaps to avoid confronting me, perhaps because of his own issues, Patrick devoted a great deal of time to his job. In fact, for all the romance, conversation and quality time that was missing from our relationship, he might as well have been deployed.

We blamed each other for our selfish pursuits and mutually allowed the growing gulf between us to continue. I felt neglected and so spent Saturday mornings running and evenings with my club friends. My husband felt ignored and coped in his own way; he stayed out late and when home, engrossed himself in computer games and I would later learn, watching pornography.

The more malnourished I became, the more hopeless my marriage felt. My health was deteriorating and my marriage was on the rocks.

Life was falling apart on so many levels.

Thirty

A Fear of Kitchens

It was somewhat ironic that I had worked at the Red Lobster Restaurant—given my fear of being around food!

In fact, I also I had an irrational fear of kitchens—the fear being, who knew what potentially uncontrollable urge to eat might come upon me while I stood so dangerously close to millions of calories?

I lived in a moment-to-moment fear that I would be unable to resist the refrigerator or the pantry. Even the word "kitchen" or "cooking" took on an evil tone; I loathed just saying the words, as if admitting that cooking instantly added fifty pounds to my body.

But getting a job was among my many plans so as to stay busy and keep out of the dangerous reach of food. Besides, my husband was busy with his own job and didn't seem to care if I was home or not.

The coffee shop appealed to me on several levels. First, I loved the location. Fountain City Coffee Shop stood along the historic Columbus Riverwalk, near the Columbus State University campus; it had an artsy feel. Within two short blocks, the Chattahoochee River pummeled boulders and wound through the ruins of an old mill. Alabama was a stone's skip away, just the opposite bank. Secondly, coffee is the nectar of the gods to an anorexic, primarily because it is calorie-free and has an amazing ability to stave off hunger for hours at a time. And another bonus: It sent me to the bathroom frequently, flushing away any extra water weight.

And as long as the shop was busy, I barely noticed the cinnamon swirled pastries and blueberry scones.

A more sinister reason I was drawn to Fountain City Coffee, was Josh.

Josh was seven years younger than me and totally not "my type." His hair was longer than mine; he had countless tattoos; and, he was a professed pagan. He had crazy hobbies like Parkour—the death-defying art of running up and down walls and hurdling obstacles like Spider-man. His rebellion tantalized me. And, he said he found me attractive.

The fact that I was married didn't stop him from his interest in pursuing a relationship with me. Afternoon shifts together became shameless four-hour flirting matches. When he put his arm around my waist, I was proud that it was so tiny. He didn't seem to notice that my collarbones jutted above the neckline of my t-shirt, or if he did, he didn't comment on it.

On a few occasions, I accepted his offer to walk down Broadway to a local brewery and have a couple beers before we went home. His hand resting on my thigh under the table felt dangerous and edgy. I justified my interest in Josh with the fact that my husband rarely touched me anymore. I blamed Patrick for that; he was too obsessed with work. Was he looking at pornography or seeing someone else? Patrick and I argued endlessly. Was I still attractive to him, or did he find me bony and repulsive? Maybe he was mad at me because due to anorexia, I could never have kids. Or maybe I was too fat. These reasons and more let me believe it was okay to accept the interest another man was showing me. Josh flirted. And I flirted back.

As long runs took up my mornings, I let slip my promise I had made to place time with the Lord ahead of my workouts. All the same, He was faithful to speak to my heart and convict me of sin. I knew my friendship with Josh was heading in a dangerous direction. The Holy Spirit leaned heavily against my heart reminding me of my commitment to my husband, "for better or worse." Even though I wasn't necessarily happy in my marriage at the moment, God still expected me to be faithful to Patrick.

I knew flirting with Josh was wrong. But while I felt God standing beside me, calling my name, and while I was terribly afraid of what would happen if I let one more thing distract my heart from Jesus, I did the unthinkable: I threw up a hand and said, "Not now, God!"

I did this knowing that He alone was keeping me alive, that He alone gave me the tiny measure of hope and peace I still had. It broke my heart that I was pushing Him away—and so I quit my job at the coffee shop. Late one afternoon, when I knew Josh wasn't working, I approached Kevin, the coffee shop manager, and said to him, "I've got to turn in my two weeks' notice."

"That's out of the blue. What's wrong? Is everything okay?" he asked.

"It's fine, the schedule's just not working out for me very well," I told him. "I'm going to start training for a marathon and I need more time in the morning for long runs."

It was half true. I was going to start training for a marathon. But the real reason was guilt. I was afraid if I did one more terrible thing, God would abandon me for good.

But though I turned away from one temptation, I walked straight back into the arms of anorexia.

Thirty-One

Race for Respect

My first marathon was the *2007 Inaugural Snickers Bar Marathon* in Albany, Georgia. Ironic, since I couldn't remember the last time I'd eaten a Snickers candy bar.

My training didn't really change. I was already logging more than 50 miles per week, running the equivalent of a marathon every Saturday morning. But somehow, like FreeWheel so many years ago, saying that I had a goal provided some legitimacy to my program.

Countless times people asked me, "Why do you run so much?"

"No reason, really," I lied over and over again. "I just love it."

What I really meant was that running made me feel like I had a reason to get up. Each morning, by the time I got home from a run, I already felt like I had conquered the world. As long as I kept this up, no one could say I didn't accomplish something.

Running also gave me a feeling of strength. Passing someone on the Riverwalk, keeping up with the guys, running three miles more than the rest of the group, confirmed in my own mind that I was strong enough not to need anyone or anything.

"I'm leaving for the race on Friday night," I told Patrick. "I'll just get a hotel for that night." We'd each been doing our own thing without regard for the other; I didn't think he'd care. "I'd rather not have to get up and drive two hours in the morning before the start."

"I was planning to go with you," he said glancing up from his computer game.

"Really?" I asked.

"Yes. I'll be done with classes on Friday by noon, so even if we leave by four o'clock, we'll get there in time for you to pick up your race packet and find a hotel."

"I had no idea you were planning to come with me." I was giddy, this felt like a real date! "Thank you!" I was so pleased that he was expressing an interest in my life.

The day of the race, my husband and I were awakened by the loud chatter of other early-rising runners gathering in the hotel hallway. Sunshine sparkled brightly and glinted off the deep puddles—all that remained of a wicked storm the night before. The fierce winds had ushered in the most exquisite race weather. Patrick and I met a few of my friends in the lobby of our hotel just before the start.

"What's your pre-race secret?" Cecil asked me. "What do you eat?"

"Nothing," I replied. "I'm always afraid it will give me a side-ache or make me sick."

"Abby, you're getting ready to run more than 26 miles, you have to eat something," Cecil said with a look of concern.

"I'll eat a little once we get going," I lied. "My stomach can handle the gels and Gatorade along the route. And I've got some snacks in my jacket pockets." By snacks, I meant 22 sugar-free hard candies with 2.5 calories a piece.

What I always found remarkable, and no doubt contributed to my not admitting to myself exactly how sick and malnourished I had become, was that so far, in all the grueling exercising and even as a long-distance runner, so far my body always performed well; my body never gave up on me. In Albany, it defied all reason once again. Even without my providing nourishment, my body powered up the hills and with enough ease to allow me to appreciate the surrounding scenery, in this case, it was difficult to miss the majestic trees towering over the lovely homes.

Families set up makeshift lemonade stands in their driveways to supplement the race's provision. One little girl kept running into the street to personally hand out orange slices to runners.

I guzzled water to keep from noticing encroaching hunger pangs; the downside being that it meant that I visited nearly every port-a-potty on the route.

"Don't stop," a spectator hollered. "There's only one woman in front of you!"

Was he talking to me? I merged back into the thinly spread sea of runners. The guy shouted again. "Hey, number one-sixty-three, you're one of the front women! Keep going, you've got this!"

I hadn't come to win—but I had come for a reason. In spite of my pride, I never set lofty goals for myself, failure hurt too much. But it couldn't hurt to kick into gear now. An unexpected win was even more impressive. So I picked up the pace, surprised that I still had energy to burn.

Two women's sneakers came into view as we passed the last mile marker. As I sailed past them, we exchanged the typical friendly rival encouragement, "Good run, keep it up."

I looked down at my thighs as I pressed a little harder. They were like chicken drumsticks, I thought: sinewy muscle clinging to knobby bone. The sight pleased me: I was burning some serious calories here.

There was one woman still in front of me. A quarter mile stretched between us. *Good run*, I told myself and let up just a little bit. I crossed the line less than three minutes after Wendy. Patrick was there to meet me. I felt like a celebrity when he smiled at me. I wondered if he was impressed.

"Come here, I want to introduce you to one of my instructors at the career course," Patrick said. "He just ran the race, too." Patrick tugged my hand after I'd caught my breath and downed a bottle of water. "CPT Edwards, this is my wife, Abby."

"Call me Dominick," he told me, "Great run! I noticed you got second female overall. Impressive! Is this your first marathon?"

"Yes." My heart swelled.

"You better pick up the pace, Kelly," Dominick said, laughing good-naturally at my husband, "or your wife is going to leave you in the dust."

Patrick and I decided not to stay for the awards ceremony. Besides, first place was recognized. But that was okay, the temporary inflation of my ego was enough.

That, and the fact that I'd earned permission from myself to eat dinner that day.

Thirty-Two

What "Problem"?

Patrick and I only expected to be stationed at Fort Benning for five months, but he accepted a second assignment there for an additional two more years.

Now without a job, and having no commitments other than the races I'd signed up for, by spring, I was restless.

Even as my mind suffered from malnutrition and overexertion, I still clamored for acceptance from others. It was important to me that others saw me as normal, going about normal activities and busy with normal things—my life, relationships and hobbies. To my way of thinking, if they saw me as normal, they would respect me.

I wanted Patrick to buy into this as well. "I think I'm going to start volunteering somewhere," I told Patrick one evening as he ate dinner in front of the TV, while I was eating my day's ration of calories: broccoli, bean sprouts, a dusting of parmesan cheese and a whole apple.

"I don't really think I should get a job right now," I told him. "Like you said, we're not going to live here very long. But I do want something to keep me occupied, to give me a sense of purpose."

"What are you thinking about doing?" he asked.

"I have an interview with the local hospice volunteer coordinator tomorrow."

"I remember the last few months of Grandpa's life, and Dad made several comments about how helpful and encouraging the hospice nurses were," I explained. "My paternal grandfather had passed away during Patrick's first deployment. "I really think that's something I can do. The schedule is flexible, it will get me out of the house and I'll be doing something good, outside of myself."

"Just don't make a bunch of weekend commitments," Patrick instructed.

His insistence infuriated me. He hardly took the effort to look at me anymore. He was always busy studying or "decompressing" with a video game. *What did he care if I never came home at all?* But I held my tongue, resolving to do whatever I wished. Besides, I doubted if he'd even notice.

The next day, I met with Michelle, the volunteer coordinator for VistaCare. Michelle was a heavyset woman with sparkling blue eyes, full cheeks and a heart bigger than Dallas.

"You'll make a perfect volunteer," Michelle said, reaching across her desk and squeezing my hand. I took in the frilly clutter of her office. The walls echoed her boisterous personality. They were papered with inspirational posters, sticky notes from her daughter declaring, "I love you," cards from hospice patients that she personally visited and a handful of notes-to-self.

"How soon can I start?"

"I love that attitude," she said grinning, and led me from her office down the hall toward a conference room. "First, I'll introduce you to the staff here, and if you're ready today, you can start watching the orientation videos."

She poked her head into each office along the hall. "Hi guys, I want to introduce you to Abby. She's our newest volunteer."

Everyone was perky and welcoming.

Even so, my mind was churning with the question, "If I admire Michelle and think she's so wonderful even though she's over weight, *Why is the fear of getting fat so debilitating?* How can I see her heart instead of her body, but I can't see past my own body well enough to determine if I have any value at all?

"There are about four hours of videos," Michelle said, popping the first VHS into the player. "They are meant to teach you how to relate to those who are dying and how to comfort the family members. It's very likely you could be visiting when someone passes, so you need to be prepared."

I'd only run eight miles that morning. My conscience berated me as I sat back into a comfy rolling chair. There was no way I was going to allow myself to sit for four hours.

"I'm sure I can't stay and watch all of them today," I told Michelle. "Is it okay if I do it over a few days and try to be ready for my first patient by next week?"

"Of course!" Michelle replied, beaming as she gently shut the conference room door behind her.

I finished the videos in four days, tapping my foot and shaking my knees constantly so as not to burn one less calorie than if I was walking around the room. When I finished, Michelle assigned me my first patient.

One of the reasons I didn't want a full-time job was because basically I could never be certain that the schedule wouldn't infringe upon my self-imposed mandatory workouts or the boss wouldn't require me to take scheduled lunch breaks. But I hadn't realized that my strict anorexic routines would complicate even a volunteer responsibility.

More than once, I had to say "no" to a last minute call from Michelle asking me to fill in for another volunteer. "I'm sorry, I'm just not available early in the morning," was a response I used quite a lot.

I became very close to the family of one of my patients. Frequently the family invited me to various celebrations, such as birthday parties, Sunday lunches and holiday gatherings. I declined every time; I was afraid to even accept her daughter Katherine's regular offer of southern sweet tea, and because Nanny lived with Katherine, a sharp-witted and very bold Christian—who took to calling me out on how thin I was.

"Abby, I'm really worried about you."

"Why?" I feigned ignorance.

"Because I've never once seen you eat. I know you run a significant number of miles every week and you look dangerously thin."

"I'm fine," I assured Katherine. "Everyone in my family is thin and running is just a hobby."

"I disagree," she countered.

What was I to say to that?

"It's not really any of my business," she continued, "but I'm afraid for you. Mother and I pray for you every night. I think you need to get some help."

Katherine was the first friend, but certainly not the last, to begin harping at me again about my low weight, my meager appetite and my obsessive workout schedule.

Soon the chorus of concern was joined by my husband's aunt, my parents, my in-laws and a few friends at church. Everyone concerned about the toll my habits had on my body.

To quiet them, to get them off my back, I told them I'd find a nutritionist and work with a counselor—which I did.

I called Remuda Ranch for a referral to local therapists. As an Alumni, I had to answer a great many questions about my current state of health.

"Honey," the staff member on the line told me, "I think your problem may be too big for you to handle on an outpatient basis."

"Please," I begged her. "Can you just give me some names? I'll think and pray about inpatient options, but I just want to start here."

"Just so you get help, now," she said, and then gave me four names, only one of whom was a female, so I called her.

"Hi," I spoke to the receptionist who had introduced herself and the clinic so fast that I wondered if I had the right place. "I'd like to make an initial appointment with Jessica S."

"When are you available?"

After we worked out the details, the receptionist reminded me to arrive early to fill out forms. I hung up the phone dazed.

Why does everyone think I have a problem?

Thirty-Three

A Divided Heart

My heart was divided, half of it owned by the people who loved me, with the other half possessed by anorexia—a most jealous and zealous paramour who consumed me.

The thing is, I was still working for approval: I longed to prove my affection for my parents, my husband and my sisters by doing this recovery thing well. I wanted to look the way they wanted me to. I wanted to eat special meals with them and participate in the daily events of their lives.

But it was hard to do that without eating.

So instead, I went to therapy as they suggested and hired a dietician. I attended group therapy, too. I hoped if everyone saw me going through the motions of getting help, they would be pleased with me. At the same time, I struggled night and day to keep from eating too much, from exercising too little, and from my irrational fears telling me I was lazy, worthless and irrelevant.

It was so difficult on the one hand, go through the motions of recovery, and at the same time choose anorexia in that I wanted, more than anything, to be slender, slim.

Gaining weight was what everyone else was telling me to do. I felt as though they were trying to change my innate self. Why couldn't they accept that this was who I was, that I was happy not eating and I enjoyed running like an Olympian?

Always in the air was the plea from others begging me to be different than what I was. I had all but forgotten what it was like to having only me setting expectation for myself. Always, always, others fielded the "Are you okay?" questions, and issued opinions, "It can't be good for you to be that thin," and directives, "You really need to get some help." On and on and on.

I forgot how to relax, to be happy and spontaneous. If I were anorexic for the rest of my life, would my family and my husband quit loving me? I didn't want to know. So I continued to please them, exhausting myself by attending treatment part-time (which appeased those who loved me) and on a full-time basis, slaving to fulfill the "to-do" list of my anorexia.

Holidays made this dichotomous behavior more difficult than usual.

"The Washburn's invited us over for the Fourth of July," my husband informed me. As usual, he told me the day before the party.

"Seriously," I asked. "You're giving me one day's notice?"

I looked at Patrick, in bed and reading, so perfect and orderly. The covers were smooth and taught over his body. With soldier-precision, he had folded them neatly under his armpits.

"I forgot."

It was obvious he had told them we would be attending.

"What time?"

"Washburn is grilling, so everyone's showing up about five."

"Am I supposed to bring anything?"

It didn't really matter whether I was supposed to bring a dish or not. I always contributed to the spread of food. What if no one else brought a veggie tray? At least by bringing my own I knew I had something that I would eat. It helped to divert suspicious questions about why I wasn't eating from the grill.

How long do you think we'll stay?" I asked Patrick nervously.

"I don't know."

"Well, can we just pick a time?" He didn't understand my anxiety and I certainly couldn't explain it to him. "How about a couple hours?"

"Probably."

It goaded me that he refused to commit. But it was just as embarrassing to admit that I couldn't handle being out of control, away from safe foods and exposed to public feasting for very long. Simply being surrounded by unlimited food choices and people eating freely continued to terrify me.

We arrived fashionably late, partly because we got lost and partly because I had a hard time deciding what to wear. Finally, I had settled on super casual jean shorts and an Old Navy t-shirt. I felt sporty and cute, but more importantly, the shirt was loose so my stomach wouldn't protrude as the night wore on and I began to feel bloated and fat—as I was sure I would even from eating just vegetables.

"Hey guys!" Washburn met us at the door with tongs in one hand and a beer in the other. "Come on in! Glad you could make it. Just set the veggie tray on the bar in the kitchen."

He led us through a small group of people, skipping formal introductions. Patrick worked with most of the guys and we wives would probably never see each other again.

Washburn's home was elaborate, made even more impressive by the fact that he'd done most of the handiwork himself. A gigantic flat screen television broadcast a 1980's Whitesnake music video through surround sound. "Fool for Your Loving," followed us through the restaurant-sized wet bar, past the glass enclosed hot tub and out onto a three-tiered, wooden deck.

"What can I get you to drink?" Washburn was a perfect host. "We have a huge selection of wine inside. I can make you any mixed drink you can think of. Or, there's a cooler of beer just behind those lawn chairs."

Patrick grabbed a Bud Light and sank into the closest chair. I felt relatively safe on the patio. Inside, on the long, tiled bar in the kitchen, was an elaborate smorgasbord, outdoors there was meat on the grill, but I couldn't see it.

"I'll have an Amstel Light," I said. Bottled beer was the best choice on these occasions. With a precise twelve ounces, it was easy to keep track of the calories.

Before long, the conversation picked up pace around me. The guys rehearsed a long week of work, talking about weapons and telling borderline dirty jokes. I retreated mentally, keeping track of their chatter enough only to laugh at the right places.

As usual, my anorexia began creating a schedule for me for the evening's activities. There are 99 calories in a beer. That means I can have two of these tonight and as many veggies as I want, but no dip, and absolutely nothing sweet.

Since I was planning on only staying a couple hours, I could spread out my food choices and drinks so that I didn't consume too many calories.

But I worried that as the night wore on, my power to resist all the delectable options would fade. If we stayed past seven, I might be tempted to have another beer, more than I had allotted calories for. So this was grounds to worry—and of course, I just start worrying now, rather than later.

Washburn was a master at the grill, turning each chicken thigh tenderly, keeping the heat low so they cooked painfully slow. It was almost seven before dinner was ready. I continued to watch Patrick, so as to make eye contact so he understood that I wanted to leave soon. But he refused to look at me.

"Hey, Babe," I spoke quietly. "We should probably go pretty soon."

"Why? I'm having a good time. I'm not ready to leave yet."

"But I am," my voice sounded whiny even to me. "I'm tired, I don't want to eat here, and you said a couple hours was okay."

Patrick never made a scene. So he tried to ignore me for a while, probably praying that like an annoying gnat I would blow away and allow him to enjoy his meal in peace.

I started to get angry, fear fueling my insistence. "Patrick, I really don't want to stay all night."

"It's the Fourth of July. The guys are talking about going to buy some really big firecrackers. Since we're outside the city limits here, we can put on our own pyrotechnic show."

"But it's barely dark," I whispered near his ear through a plastered smile. "That will be hours from now."

He didn't answer. I noticed Washburn glance our way and pretend not to notice our hushed argument. Patrick saw it, too.

"Look, just let me finish eating and I'll take you home."

"Really?"

"Yes, but I'm coming back."

"But..." I started to protest then realized that I had won as much ground as he would permit me. It was a compromise. He wouldn't insist that I stay and pretend to have a good time, but he wasn't going to let me ruin his time with friends, either.

"Hey man," Patrick addressed Washburn, who was scrubbing the grill. "I'm going to take Abby home. She's not feeling great, but I'll be back. Don't start the pyro show without me!"

The first half of the drive home was quiet. It wasn't a short trip, the silence hung oppressively.

"Thanks for taking me home. I really need to eat something."

Patrick pretended to watch the road intently.

"I don't understand," he finally muttered. "Why couldn't you just eat there? Why can't you just hang out like a normal person?"

He was right. I knew that my attempts to be normal and anorexic at the same time were failing. I simply couldn't share my life with others, and still devote my life to anorexia. I truly couldn't love my husband and become one with him while selling my soul to an eating disorder as predatory as anorexia.

Patrick pulled up in front of our apartment. I slid out of the truck and stood in the open door frame for just a second. I tried to look at my husband and smile. "Thanks," I said again.

He didn't answer me, just reached across the seat and pulled the passenger door closed. As he pulled away, he waved—an indication that he wasn't furious with me. He was confused, hurt and at a loss as to how to help his wife.

By the time he made it back to Washburn's, it would be pitch dark, the perfect time for putting on a spectacular Fourth of July fireworks show. But in as much as it would have been a lovely thing to share together, once again, my anorexia had claimed that part of my heart, taking me away from those who loved me best.

Thirty-Four

A Different Kind of Cheating

For most of my life, I'd felt like the screw-up in a sea of mostly perfect people. I was the reason my parents worried and couldn't sleep at night. I was the one who cost them and my grandparents thousands upon thousands of dollars for counseling sessions and treatment centers. And it was me who failed at making sure their hard-earned money paid off; even with all the time, effort and hope spent on "curing Abby" none had been successful. I was the reason one of my sisters had nightmares about death. I was the reason my husband would never have a son or daughter.

The more these realities registered within my head and heart, the exacerbated my condition became. *Why bother to eat if I was a problem, an inconvenience, a burden, an expense, a cause for fear, second best, expendable?*

Wasn't anorexia simply a slow route to suicide?

Why was everyone else perfect, and I wasn't?

And then, about seven years into marriage, I discovered that my husband wasn't perfect either. He had his own issues with faithfulness, his own divided loyalties. The betrayal hurt, but in a strange way it was relieving.

I struggled to extend to Patrick the same understanding and compassion for his failures as my family had shown me in my addiction to an eating disorder

Instead, hurt and angered by his indiscretion, I used his sin as leverage for my own pride. At least I hadn't done what he did. For once, I wasn't the only person who didn't measure up, who wasn't perfect. I used this information against him; he became the scapegoat for my relapse. I let him take the fall for our disintegrating relationship.

By the time we changed duty stations from Georgia to Washington, I had one foot out the door. But as usual, God's timing is perfect. Just when I felt I'd lost everything, God brought back to me a great treasure and comfort that I had set aside.

During the last year we lived in Georgia, I had finally gotten a job. While I loved working at Barnes and Noble, the mandatory weekends and occasional late nights whittled away what little time I had reserved for my husband.

One night as the store neared closing time, I was collecting stray magazines around the cafe. My eyes fell on a title I hadn't noticed before, Writer's Digest. Something about it piqued my interest. I had once been an avid writer, especially in the private pages of my journal. But as anorexia took over my imagination, I had stopped writing. But seeing the copy of Writer's Digest made me recall how much I liked to write, and how it inspired me.

I remembered Proverbs 16:24 *"Pleasant words are like a honeycomb, sweetness to the soul and health to the body."*

The next morning, I began to write being reminded by that Writer's Digest magazine and how much I enjoyed perusing the articles.

FINDING MY PEN AND MY VOICE
Of my brutal iron cage.
Transfixed and frozen by starvation's ugly stare.
Hunger held my voice, the key,
Dangled it outside my cage.
Hunger glanced and silence,
They laughed maliciously.
BUT JUST LAST NIGHT, SOMETHING HAPPENED!
Through course, conviction, and conversation.
The world seemed so much bigger,
Than my silent, metal cage.
The gnawing deep inside, gave way to simple rage.
I WANT MY VOICE, I NEED MY PEN!
There's so much I want to say.
And somehow as I screamed these words,
The bars crumbled and decayed.
Silence screamed in pain!
The key clattered toward my cage,
I grasped my pen, began again and put my voice to page.

It was the first of many things I would write.

The next month I began writing my blog, which I aptly named, *Predatory Lies*, which emanated from my desire to discuss with others the relentless, insidious lies that I knew controlled my own life. I hoped that exposing them would help loosen their powerful hold over me. Perhaps by admitting them publicly, I could lessen the shame I felt, and better come to terms over how guilty I felt for the burden I'd been to my family. If nothing else, I hoped that others affected by eating disorders would find hope and healing in my words.

I began to use the blog as my journal, sharing nearly everything that came to mind. Much of what I wrote was poetry and prayer concerning my own hope to live, and to live a purpose-driven life.

I strived to share the love of Jesus in my posts.

The more I wrote, I was surprised by the joy creeping into and seeping out of my words.

Even as I began to share, confront and refute the lies of anorexia, my marriage continued to crumble. This too, offered rich material to share with my readers, telling them about the loneliness and pain I felt in my marriage. *"He ignored my birthday, watches television constantly instead of talking to me. He never even looks at me, let alone makes eye contact. I'm afraid that his apathy and ignoring me is making the anorexia even worse. We need counseling, but if I tell him, he will be angry. I don't know what to do. Right now I find myself vying for his attention, but I know performing for others triggers my eating disorder. Constantly trying to please him makes me feel unworthy and I blame him. But is that really his fault?"*

Readers identified with my issues, thanked me for revealing them and offered advice. Later, I wrote in my journal:

"I journaled online yesterday about Patrick and got an interesting response. Someone said that he's not off the hook, his issues are real and need to be dealt with, but as much as his emotional and sometimes physical abandonment triggers me, anorexia is obviously my significant other. It's as if I've been cheating on him, having an affair, effectively isolating and ignoring Patrick."

The blog was therapeutic, like a droplet of hope from Heaven. God was using my husband's infidelity to illumine His grace for me—and asking that I seek forgiveness in my own life.

Was God using a dying marriage to rescue a starving girl—a girl He loved so very much?

Thirty-Five

Divorce?

Ten months later, in August 2008, the Army moved us to Fort Lewis, Washington. More literally, they moved me. Patrick had to stay in Georgia an extra month to wrap up his job there and hand over the reins to his successor. So, I flew into Seattle late one beautiful afternoon, hustled to our new home and signed the mortgage papers.

Before I left Georgia, Patrick and I discussed my condition, and whether it was appropriate timing for me to seek help with my eating disorder and return to an inpatient treatment program.

"I just don't feel like now is the right time for me to go inpatient," I told him. "You're going to deploy from your new unit. I can't just take off and go to the hospital for however long. Someone needs to take care of the new house and keep things running while you're gone."

"Abby, there's never going to be a 'right' time," he argued. "Even your parents say you look almost as bad as you did in college. My aunt Cindy even commented that she's worried about you. You have to get some kind of help."

"I will," I promised. "I'll find an outpatient counselor and a dietician, too. But there's nothing they can tell me that I don't already know. I just need to do what I know I must do to get better. I can do this myself."

Maybe it was the fact that Patrick would soon be deploying for a year. Maybe it was all the abuse my heart had already suffered between his emotional abandonment and my destructive relationship with anorexia. Maybe it was the new energy I felt from connecting with others via the blog.

Whatever it was, as soon as I arrived in Washington I got a job working at Starbucks and quickly began to meet new friends. Without Patrick at home and the constant pain of feeling ignored, replaced by a video game or a movie, I felt less lonely. I even contemplated divorce—something I had believed from the core of my being would never happen to me. I was raised to believe that divorce was never, ever acceptable. But I didn't think I could stay in this marriage.

I began contacting divorce lawyers with questions.

Patrick arrived mid-September, and when he did, our marriage completely fell apart.

I asked Patrick why he married me, if he would rather look at provocative pictures, or simply play his video games all the time. He told me, "I married for stability."

I begged him to tell me if he really loved me. Did he love me as much of he loves his games and time to himself?

"About the same," he had said.

This realization created a pain so great that I didn't think I could endure it.

With great trepidation, I called my parents. More than fearful of their response, I felt so awful admitting that once again I had failed. Gosh, would I always be the problem child to them? After all the anxiety I had caused them over my health, now I was calling with a failed marriage, begging them to help me one more time.

Mercifully, and without judgment, Dad put my mom on a flight to Seattle the very next weekend. In the meantime, I quit my job at Starbucks and began to collect boxes and price U-Haul trailers.

The night before my mother arrived to drive back to Kansas with me, I told Patrick that I was leaving.

"You do what you have to do," he replied without looking at me. "I'm not going to chase you."

I went to bed crushed; he never came to bed.

The next morning I slipped past him asleep in his chair. Hugging my gym bag close to my chest, I slipped into the garage. The door creaked painfully as it opened behind me and I backed out. I didn't want to wake him; the last thing I wanted was to see my husband.

It was Sunday, which used to be my one day of rest from working out. But I went anyway.

What shouldn't have been a workout at all, morphed from a quick jog on the treadmill to a full-fledged Crossfit™ training session. Anger and hurt roiled in me. I remember thinking that if my heart seized suddenly from over exertion, it wouldn't be the worst thing.

Maybe if I died here on the gym floor someone would call my husband and perhaps they might see some flicker of compassion or loss on his face.

Mom's plane didn't arrive in Seattle until five in the evening. That left hours before I needed to pick her up, hours to avoid going home.

I climbed into the car, freshly showered and punched the radio. The Christian station reminded me that it was Sunday morning. An hour at church couldn't hurt.

There was a fledgling church nearby, just off Marvin Road. The congregation was so young that they were still meeting in the cafeteria of a local elementary school. My coworker, Clifton, and his wife were the only two people I knew there, so it seemed a safe place to hover in the shadows as the hours passed.

I pulled into the parking lot and flipped open my phone. It buzzed an email alert. Patrick. I debated whether to read it. Finally, I scrolled down to the single sentence. "Please don't leave."

Fury raged through me. How could he be so heartless, so disconnected that even as I was about to leave him, he couldn't look me in the eyes and ask me to stay? Tossing my phone under the front seat, I went inside the church.

Praise music ebbed and flowed around me. The sound of simple guitars, quiet melodies, and familiar words flooded my ears. "While I'm Waiting," by John Waller was the third song.

"I'm waiting
I'm waiting on You, Lord and I am hopeful
I'm waiting on You, Lord though it is painful
But patiently, I will wait
I will move ahead, bold and confident taking every step in obedience
While I'm waiting I will serve You
While I'm waiting
I will worship
While I'm waiting I will not faint
I'll be running the race
Even while I wait
I'm waiting
I'm waiting on You, Lord
And I am peaceful
I'm waiting on You, Lord
Though it's not easy
But faithfully, I will wait."

That's me, Lord, I thought. *Only I'm not waiting patiently.*

I was stuck in a vicious limbo between the painful familiar and a scary future. I was used to restricting food and enduring intense exercise. I was use to living lonely in the cocoon of intimacy with anorexia.

But I'm waiting, like a pendulum hanging in midair between that place and a tempting freedom. What would it feel like not to think about calories and workouts? What would it feel like not to try and make my husband love me?

I wanted a clean break from everything that ever hurt me. I wanted to be free from anorexia and free from my husband. Maybe one change would precipitate the other.

And God it's true, here in the midst of waiting, I want to serve you. I want to find comfort in belonging to you. I need your peace.

The sermon was lost to me. I don't remember any of it. For the entire hour, I was mesmerized by the couple in front of me, their fingers intertwined, so that I could barely tell where his hand ended and hers began. Will that ever be me? I wondered what it felt like.

The Holy Spirit will use any means to capture our hearts and woo us toward Him. The music continued to weave its way between my anxieties, softening my earlier anger.

New truths, and those long ignored wafted on the harmonies. Like a fresh butterfly, my heart opened. Grace and humility flowed in. Suddenly, my heart would clamp closed, as if the chill of unfamiliar wisdom startled me and was almost too much to bear. I wonder if a butterfly ever considered crawling back into its cocoon.

What if I didn't leave? In many ways, staying seemed the easier thing to do, like cuddling back up into my familiar problem, my familiar role of being the sick one, of focusing only on how much I exercised and how little I ate, instead of on a more scary problem, my failing marriage.

I slipped out the back of the makeshift sanctuary during the final prayer, hoping to miss the chummy farewells and well wishes. Darn, I thought, as Clifton found me in the parking lot.

"Hey, Abby, how are you?" He took a closer look at my face and asked, "What's wrong?"

What would he think? Would he see me as a strong, self-reliant woman if I told him I was leaving my husband? Or would he deem me a failure? What did it even matter?

"I'm leaving my husband," I told him.

"Oh, Abby. I'm so sorry."

Clifton promised to pray for us.

When I got home, I didn't go into the living room. The noise from Patrick's television show droned above me.

I need to start packing, I thought. My home workout room was in the basement. I decided to start there, culling out the most important things to take with me. But soon I was overwhelmed. I sat on the floor surrounded by a half dozen boxes, my lap laden with fitness DVDs, a tangled jump rope lay at my feet.

What if leaving didn't change anything? Patrick and I had spent almost ten years together. How would I ever separate what was me and mine without destroying both of us?

My cell phone rang; it was Mom calling from Denver. "Hey, hon. Everything's on time. I just wanted you to know that I'm praying for you and Patrick constantly, and I'll see you in about three hours.

"Okay," I cried. "Mom, I don't know where to begin. I can't even think clearly enough to pack. What am I doing? What am I going to do?"

"Don't do anything, Sweetheart." Mom's voice was comforting. "I'll help you when I get there. Just hang on."

When I hung up with Mom, I stood, scattering everything from my lap. Climbing the stairs felt like battling a down elevator. My feet were heavy, disconnected stumps. At the main level of the house, I peeked around the corner into the living room where Patrick still sat. He was playing a game by then, thumbs flipping and jerking as his avatar raced to rescue the princess.

I wished that he would chase me like that. I muttered and my anger at him flared again. Making my way to our bedroom on the top floor was just as difficult as the first flight of stairs. Finally, I sank to my knees and crawled the last few steps, tears falling from my eyes. My stomach clenched.

Did he ever love me? Why can't he love me? What's wrong with me?

In the master bathroom, I sat cross-legged before my set of cabinets. Of course I had to take my blow dryer, my deodorant and shampoo. I could pack this part without too much thought. A shadow in the doorway caught the corner of my eye.

"I don't want you to leave." Patrick said, leaning halfway into the bathroom as if something invisible kept him from coming any closer to me. His eyes were watery, but he never cried. I stared at him, unblinking, unnerved and mute.

"I need you to stay."

In a fraction of a second, a scene from 15 years earlier flashed through my mind. Daddy and I stood in the garage hanging up our coats and aligning our muddy boots after feeding the dogs in the rain.

"Abby, I don't know what else to do," he had said. "I don't know how to help you. All of your promises to gain weight haven't happened. I'm frustrated and your mom and I are tired. You are going to have to go back to the hospital."

"Please, Daddy, please no. Give me just one more chance. Can I just have until Thanksgiving? Please don't give up on me, just one more chance."

Fear laced my words. I'd give anything not to face the feeling of abandonment one more time, having to watch my family walk away, leaving me in the hands of doctors and dietitians.

Now, years later, I knew what Dad had felt. A surge of compassion, an unparalleled hope, a fiery love that always protects, trusts, hopes and perseveres. But Dad had reached out and drew me into his chest.

"I love you so much," he whispered into my hair. "You know I will never, ever leave you. I only want you to live."

Now, from the other side of that equation, I looked up into the eyes of another man. I understood Daddy's heart.

I stood, leveling my eyes to Patrick's. "Do you really want me? Do you really need me?"

He nodded. I put my hand in his and let him draw me into his chest.

"If you want me, if you swear you really need and love me, I will never leave you.

"I cannot live constantly wondering if I'm important to you. You have to learn to show me that you love me."

"God has given me so many hundreds of chances despite my rebellion and failures. I'm so far from perfect and have made so many of the same mistakes hundreds of times. But I can't receive that grace and not extend it too."

We continued to stand in the bathroom, silent.

That afternoon, I accepted a purpose, a calling, God's intention for my life. I was to be this man's helpmate, his completer.

I must be in this marriage to do that.

I must be alive in order to do that.

Thirty-Six

So Many Second Chances

Patrick and I moved into the hallway and sank onto the top stair. We faced the octagon window that peeked out from the second floor. The window captured a bird's eye view below us. Neighbor children were playing kickball; Brian, next-door neighbor was forever watering his lawn. Our hearts were transforming, our worlds rewinding and resetting, and no one even paused.

Mom's plane was in the air even as we sat there silent. Finally, I stood first. "I have to pick up my mom at the airport."

"What are you going to tell her?"

"That I'm staying. Other than that, what can I say?"

I knew what he was asking. How could things ever be the same? It would be hard enough to go on together, waking each morning, forcing ourselves not to remember what almost happened. But even if we could manage a fresh perspective, how could we expect those who loved us to simply pretend that nothing ever happened?

I drove through the maze of Seattle's airport, parked and found my way to baggage claim without getting lost. For those few spare minutes before Mom deplaned, I leaned against a concrete pillar, just breathing. Before too long, I saw the face of the person I so love, coming toward me. I broke into a grin.

"Mom!" I ran toward her as if I wasn't nearly 30 years old.

"Hey, Sweetheart." Mom dropped her carryon and hugged me.

Mom always smells good with a combination of lingering perfume, coconut-scented shampoo and my dad's aftershave still clinging to her cheek from his goodbye kiss. She wore one of her signature jackets to ward off the traveler's chill. This one was denim, stylishly cuffed at the sleeves revealing a coordinating shirt beneath. And of course, her shoes were the perfect complement, earthy sandals the exact same true red as her shirt.

"You look cheerier than I expected," she smiled at me and held me at arm's length.

"Well, I have some good news for you. At least, I hope you think it's good since you've already flown out here." I took a deep breath. "Mom, I'm not leaving Patrick. God is breaking through and I think He's going to save us."

I never should have wondered how I was going to live the next days, weeks and months. I never should have worried about how my parents would react. For the next three days, those days she had allotted to help me pack and move home, Mom became God's living example of forgiveness, grace and hundredth chances.

Mom and I loaded her suitcase in my car and began the hour drive to my home. She never asked a probing question about the miracle that transpired while she was high in the sky aboard the airplane. Instead, she asked only what we were going to do together for the next couple days.

Patrick was at the house when we got home. They hugged.

As we went to bed that night, I thanked God for parents who still loved me, who hadn't abandoned me after 17 years of consistent failure, expensive treatments and so much heartache. Parents who would still come to my rescue after so many years of seeming futile efforts to save me from myself.

I started to see how similar the situations of my eating disorder and my crumbling marriage were. Perhaps God used those years as a painful training ground for my parents, so that when they were called upon to teach their children about God's expansive forgiveness and unconditional grace that they would be prepared to live it out.

Many, many times during my battle with anorexia, I tried to convince my parents that I had gained the upper hand—that the war's tide was turning in my favor. In reality, I only wanted to placate them so they would leave me to my own devices.

I recall expecting their accolades and high praise for eating a single piece of pizza. "See, don't you see? I did it! Why won't you get off my back about eating more?"

In much the same way, Patrick wanted me to accept a single peck on the cheek, or his foot touching mine beneath the covers as proof of his affection for me. "I touched you last night," he would say. "Why are you complaining that I'm not affectionate?"

Another similarity between Patrick and me, was that for many years I complained he had abandoned me emotionally and even physically, yet I refused to admit that basically, I had already emotionally left him.

Countless conversations were moot, as I tallied calories in my head while he spoke to me. He pulled away sexually but I had already manipulated my body into prepubescent form and often shied away from him in shame over my body. Truthfully, if he had asked me to choose between him and my eating disorder, I would have chosen anorexia.

For the first several years, I denied that I needed help. Even amidst the concern of those who knew me best, I wanted to believe I was okay and could find the solution to my eating disorder on my own. Patrick too, wanted to believe that if he just tried harder, he could avoid pornographic websites and learn to be vulnerable and intimate with his own wife.

As for me, anorexia robbed me of all ability to create and live within meaningful relationships. An eating disorder builds a shell around its victim, fending off anyone whose love might threaten it.

How long had my parents endured my rejection of their love, the extension of their help, the sincerity of their prayers and encouragement? How long had Patrick selfishly engaged in shallow, secondary forms of sexual fulfillment while avoiding me? Just how different were we?

Mom spent those next few days with us, loving us in spite of ourselves and in the middle of our mess. Christ-like, she never condemned or advised a list of right behaviors that might somehow accomplish salvation for our marriage. At the same time, she walked beside me again, just as she had done in the lowest point of my anorexia.

Without so much as a word, Mom led me closer to the Savior whose irrevocable love would save my life again, and this time, redeem my marriage.

Three days later, we purchased a flight back to Kansas for Mom. I could have spent a year marinating in and absorbing her faith, compassion and joy. Oh for that Christ-likeness to fill me up and overflow into my marriage!

Thirty-Seven

Recovery—and a New Beginning

As I write this last chapter, I am grateful for what feels like a second chance at life.

For almost five years, I've lived a new life, drastically changed from my years with anorexia. I am learning to ride the wax and wane of life; that is the best indicator of my full recovery. I can accept, endure and learn to enjoy change. I can live outside of routine. I can pull up stakes, when the army says "move," spend 40 hours in the car and set up house on the opposite coast without starving myself. I can face new things without reverting to old behaviors.

Just a few moments ago, I clicked "accept changes" on this imposing document that is my life story on paper. With the release of a button, much of the old was undone and replaced with tighter prose and smoother transitions. I needed to make specific changes. Looking at the manuscript now, I don't miss what is gone because it was replaced by something much better.

Similarly, anorexia was deleted from my life line by line. But each terrifying deletion has been replaced with a more healthy habit, a grander experience and brighter hope.

This has been true for each of the major issues. Most changes have seemed to overtake me by accident. I turn around and suddenly realize I no longer have any interest in the limited horizon and the confining rituals of anorexia. As I watch other people dig into lives of maybe's and mess-ups and momentary whims, I am fascinated. In embracing change I am, as C. S. Lewis says, "Surprised by joy."

For starters, I thought it would kill me to change my habit of running. In fact, as I regained my health, I toyed with the idea of hanging onto that one thing, trying to morph it into a healthier version of my previous obsession. I got my dog, Brave, four years ago during Patrick's third deployment. We started taking long walks together. In the course of time I discovered I was not running anymore.

My perception of food has changed slowly, but pleasantly. It still tickles me when I pick up peppermint mocha coffee creamer and toss it thoughtlessly into my cart. It isn't fat-free or the lowest calorie option. Even so, my mouth waters with anticipation for my "morning joe." I smile to myself when I taste the samples offered at the grocery store or steal a sip of my husband's chocolate shake from McDonald's, and I don't count the French fries-freedom has emerged.

An equally important counterpart to personal change IS allowing others to change, and willingness to wait, wait, and wait for that to happen. Sometimes, it means accepting others when they refuse to change.

Marriage is the proving ground for all kinds of character development. One of my favorite Bible study teachers said, "God didn't give you a spouse to make you happy, he gave you a spouse to make you holy."

My struggle with anorexia infused me with grace and patience for my husband. Indeed, in the course of eleven years, some of his hurtful behaviors haven't changed yet. It is difficult for him to show affection or to experience emotional intimacy, and sometimes I think things will never change.

There's a great deal of tension between "never", "maybe", and "someday", and change can occur in any one of these places. I know that God can take a recalcitrant heart, like mine trapped by the lies of anorexia, still screaming, "never", and allow change to mysteriously overtake it. I have been in that place of, "maybe I want things to be different but I'm not sure how." Today I'm walking in the illumination of "someday", letting God change my heart day by day and trusting him to work in Patrick's heart too.

I am finally at my ideal weight. Not because I have any idea what the scale would say, but because I am truly happy—healthy and capable of enjoying my life to the fullest.

Yes, I have absolutely gained weight since my days of anorexia, but I have no idea how much or what the number is. I do know that at this weight, my arms are strong, my hair and fingernails are growing. I'm not cold all the time. If you hug me, you won't be able to count my ribs. I can eat birthday cake and pumpkin pie on Thanksgiving. I'm not scared or anxious anymore. That alone is worth the weight.

As I gained weight, my brain began to function normally and rationally again.

No longer constantly obsessed with my food and body, I redirected my self-discipline into a determination to be grateful for my body, using it to honor God and bless others.

Finally, I can see outside of myself, outside of the chaos in my head. Recently, Brave and I got certified as a pet therapy team. Several times a week, we go into hospitals, nursing homes, schools and even homes for abused children. There, we get to help them find joy and respite from the hurt and struggles in their own lives.

My relationships with my parents and sisters have changed drastically, too. I treasure the deep friendship that I have with my mother, now that she is no longer in constant fear of losing me. Dad painstakingly edited this book with me. What a joy to relive the memories and know it is our past, to feel the sadness of our story and know that God has redeemed it. My heart soars when one of my sisters calls me for advice, implying that once again she sees me as her big sister.

Finally, I believe I'm beautiful. Someone asked me recently to describe how a godly woman pursues beauty. I couldn't answer. For a while, I'd tried to override my desire for personal beauty. The pursuit of attractiveness can be deadly.

But, being personally created in the image of God, it's impossible to discount God's appreciation for beauty. The Bible talks about beautiful women: Abigail, Bathsheba, Sarah, Rebekah, Rachel and Esther were all described as beautiful women. Psalm 45:11 says, "The king is enthralled by your beauty; honor Him, for He is your Lord."

And Ecclesiastes 3:11 says, "Yet God has made everything beautiful for its own time. He has planted eternity in the human heart, but even so, people cannot see the whole scope of God's work from beginning to end."

God is the author of beauty and wants me to enjoy it.

And I now make friends easily, and the friendships are lasting, meaningful and important to me.

The Army continues to shuffle my husband and me around to various duty stations on both coasts. But now, instead of turning inward, fearing loneliness and finding comfort in an eating disorder, I allow God to introduce me to some of His beautiful women. I find my own reflection in them.

While we were stationed in Washington, I met Dana. She quickly became the best friend I've ever had. Her husband deployed with Patrick and for a season, we acted like two sisters. Dana was a living, breathing example of the kind of freedom I longed for. Her relationship with food and exercise seemed so refreshing and uncomplicated. She was a healthy weight and she devoured life and relished food.

Though we were both Christians and had known Jesus for most of our lives, Dana exuded an understanding of grace and freedom in Christ that I wasn't experiencing.

As my friendship with Dana deepened, I began to let go of my demonic dance partner—anorexia. I found myself reaching toward the hand of my Savior.

Alive to life and aware of others, I have no shortage of friends. We run the usual gamut of conversation about our insecurities. I look across the table and enjoy their friendships, and soak up their joy and happiness. We share memories and hopes. We talk of children and pets and the struggles of marriage. Our hearts melt together, and we find the true meaning of friend.

"Abby, you are so beautiful," I hear. "You glow. You're radiant. Your skin looks bright; your eyes are lively. Something about you is just beautiful."

Finally, I can say it. I am beautiful. And why shouldn't I be? I am God's creation.

God began beautifying me from the inside. From the inside to the outside, He is building my confidence, humility, beauty, appreciation and wisdom.

The Bible says that Jesus grew in wisdom, in stature and in favor with God and man. I want to grow that way too: physically, mentally and spiritually. May all these facets of our many-sided beings be beautiful to Him.

And, I can now find peace in the eye of any storm. Yesterday I stood beneath a store's canopy during a violent thunderstorm. I'd run into Michael's—the arts and craft store, and just as I was checking out, the sky ripped open and began to pour. Taking my change, I went outside and huddled on the sidewalk under a short overhang. There I looked on in wonder and great amazement as God directed a glorious symphony in nature.

Thunder provided percussion and tiny raindrops played a rhythmic melody. Once motionless trees whipped back and forth as the wind threw up a magnificent spray. Almost instantly, I was drenched head to toe despite the shelter. Mist like that of a monstrous ocean wave washed my face.

I had places to be. I needed to pick up the dog from the groomer, head home to make dinner and finish an article I'm working on, but for almost a half hour, I leaned back against the rough brick building, as I chose to simply be in the storm.

For me, there is something about nature that evokes praise. I began to thank God for many things, but specifically, in that moment, for healing me of anorexia and reintroducing me to true beauty. Thunder rolled in successive rumbles. It sounded like Almighty God answering me, assuring me of His complete control over my life—and over the entire world.

In a quiet dawning, against the backdrop of the storm, God began to show me how much he has been changing the inside of me as much as the outside. Not so many years ago this storm would have made me afraid. Not of thunder and lightning, but of deeper, anxious things.

As the storm raged, the temperature dropped ten degrees. In the past, I was too thin, with no fat to insulate my body. There's no way I could have thoroughly enjoyed this moment.

Rainy days used to make me fretful about the next morning's run. How could I get in a long workout to burn enough calories if it was pouring rain?

When anorexia controlled my mind and choices, I was unable to think of anything except food and exercise. Even in the midst of this beautiful storm, I would have fretted over what was for dinner, if I'd worked out hard enough that day, or how many calories were in the string cheese I ate before I left the house.

We know that God longs to shape us into the image of His Son, Jesus Christ, but that doesn't change the very real beauty of our mortality.

I have no purchase in tomorrow. I have no power over yesterday. But in this one, singular moment, I can find God and enjoy the beauty of His love for me, evidenced in creation, especially His intimate creation of me.

"I will give thanks to you because I have been so amazingly and miraculously made. Your works are miraculous, and my soul is fully aware of this" (Psalms 139:14).

"Return to your rest, my soul, for the Lord has been good to you" (Psalm: 116:7).

Book Clubs Questions for Discussion and Reflection

1. Abby's particular eating disorder was diagnosed as anorexia. Do you have a family member or friend who may have an eating disorder? What makes you think so, and what have you done about it so far? What else can you do to help, or can you?

2. Though Abby's family picked up on her deterioration fairly early, at what point did Abby herself become concerned? Describe a time when someone came to you because they were genuinely worried about you. Who was that person and what concern did he or she have? Describe a time when you were genuinely worried about yourself—and what you did about it?

3. Abby's parents were assertive in addressing her eating disorder and because she was a minor, they were able to insist that she get treatment. Do you think her parents handled the situation correctly? Did they allow her to try to get well on her own for too long (bargaining, setting weight goals, bribing her with a German shepherd), or did they force her to get help too early? How do you know when it's time to get help?

4. In the early stages of her disorder, Abby felt that one way to make others like her more and see her as a disciplined person was to be thin—and so she began to restrict her food intake and do physical activities with the goal of burning calories. When you look in the mirror, what "image" do you see? Describe the relationship you have with "the face in the mirror." Are you happy with the "relationship" you have with yourself? What is one thing about that person in the mirror would you like to change—and how would you change it? In looking at your reflection, whose opinion of that person matters most—yours, or that of others?

5. In reading Abby's account of her battle to overcome anorexia, at what point did it become clear to you that for all of Abby's attempts to "do

better at getting better," she had lost control of her free will and that her disease had taken over and was ruling her mind? What is free will? Do you have a habit or admitted addiction such as caffeine or smoking? Describe it. How can you tell when you have lost "free will"—and that your "habit" has morphed into an addiction?

6. Abby tells this story from her own point of view, but mentions how deeply her family members were affected. Describe an action or aspect of your own life that positively or negatively affects those closest to you. Why do you think our actions have such broad consequences?

7. There's a saying, "We don't live in a vacuum." What do you think that means? Describe a time when you have been personally hurt by someone else's actions. How did you deal with that? Did you confront them? How did they respond? Regardless of their response, what can you do to protect yourself? Should you stay in that relationship?

8. Abby said that "Marriage is the proving ground for all kinds of character development." What do you think she means by this? If you are married or in a long-term relationship, what are some ways that you have been forced to compromise, or change, in order to make the relationship work for the both of you? If you are not married, what other relationship(s) has effect change in your life, good or bad?

9. Some of Abby's behaviors, such as lying, suicidal tendencies and hurtful exaggerations, ("You will never see me again...") are common among those dealing with eating disorders and are key indicators of a problem. Have you had any of these symptoms, or noticed any of these in a loved one? What can you do, and who can you turn to for help? Have you admitted to yourself, or others, that you believe you have an eating disorder? If so, what happened next? How are you now?

10. In what way did Abby's eating disorder complicate the troubles in her marriage? In what way did her recovery improve the couple's relationship?

11. In the preface, Tamara Pryor explains the prevalence and severity of eating disorders in modern society. In what way do you see evidence of this within your local high school or church or the community at large? In your opinion, how prevalent is anorexia in the country as a whole?

12. What do you think were the primary factors in Abby developing an eating disorder? Do you think the media plays a role in how we see ourselves in relationship to body image, and if so, how is that best mitigated?

13. What is your sense of "how" an eating disorder begins? After reading Abby's book, and in looking at Abby's timeline of her eating disorder, from onset to recovery, how has your notion of anorexia changed?

14. Abby alludes to the fact her eating disorder possibly had origin when she felt pressure from family and peers for not being "enough." In her quest for a greater sense of personal power, she concludes "I'll be 'more,' but it will be on my terms." From this new self-awareness to "make change," she targets her body as the agent to show others that she is disciplined and focused. She sets out to restrict her food intake and adheres to an extreme schedule of exercise. While others close to Abby see a person who is dangerously thin, Abby in fact, derives a sense of personal achievement from obsessively controlling her weight through diet and exercise. In what way do see this "reasoning" as to why eating disorders get a psychiatric listing?

ABOUT THE AUTHOR

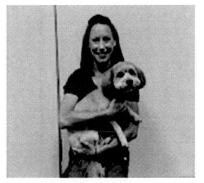

Abby Kelly is an author and blogger on the topic of eating disorder awareness, prevention, and treatment. Abby writes passionately about her 15-year battle with anorexia, including three inpatient stays and many years of outpatient counseling, and how she finally got free.

Her outreach to others includes those struggling with other eating disorders. Abby's blog, *Predatory-Lies* and has millions of followers. Her work in the field of eating disorders has been published in *Haven Journal, She Loves Magazine, Start Marriage Right* and Believer Life. She is the managing editor as well as a contributor to FINDINGbalance's blog.

Abby is an active member of the FaithWriter's community, and has led numerous Bible studies at local churches, through Protestant Women of the Chapel and currently through an online program called Good Morning Girls.

Abby is married to an officer in the US Army. Abby and her dog, Brave, are certified as a therapy team through Pet Partners, and enjoy visiting patients in hospitals and nursing homes as well as helping children practice reading both at school and in local libraries.

To contact the author to speak to your group or for more information, visit: www.predatory-lies.com

APPENDIX A: Clinical Information about Anorexia

Anorexia Nervosa is a serious, potentially life-threatening eating disorder characterized by self-starvation and excessive weight loss.

The following information is a brief summary of the Feeding and Eating Disorders described in the American Psychiatric Association's Fifth Edition of the Diagnostic and Statistical Manual of Mental Disorders (DSM-5), published in 2013.

About Anorexia Nervosa:
- Approximately 90-95% of anorexia Nervosa sufferers are girls and women.
- Between 0.5–1% of American women suffer from anorexia Nervosa.
- Anorexia Nervosa is one of the most common psychiatric diagnoses in young women.
- Between 5-20% of individuals struggling with anorexia Nervosa will die. The probabilities of death increases within that range depending on the length of the condition.
- Anorexia Nervosa has one of the highest death rates of any mental health condition.
- Anorexia Nervosa typically appears in early to mid-adolescence.

Symptoms:
- Inadequate food intake leading to a weight that is clearly too low.
- Intense fear of weight gain, obsession with weight and persistent behavior to prevent weight gain.
- Self-esteem overly related to body image.
- Inability to appreciate the severity of the situation.
- Binge-Eating/Purging Type involves binge eating and/or purging behaviors during the last three months.
- Restricting Type does not involve binge eating or purging.
- Eating disorders experts have found that prompt intensive treat-

ment significantly improves the chances of recovery. Therefore, it is important to be aware of some of the warning signs of anorexia Nervosa.

Warning Signs:
- Dramatic weight loss.
- Preoccupation with weight, food, calories, fat grams, and dieting.
- Refusal to eat certain foods, progressing to restrictions against whole categories of food (e.g. no carbohydrates, etc.).
- Frequent comments about feeling "fat" or overweight despite weight loss.
- Anxiety about gaining weight or being "fat."
- Denial of hunger.
- Development of food rituals (e.g. eating foods in certain orders, excessive chewing, rearranging food on a plate).
- Consistent excuses to avoid mealtimes or situations involving food.
- Excessive, rigid exercise regimen--despite weather, fatigue, illness, or injury, the need to "burn off" calories taken in.
- Withdrawal from usual friends and activities.
- In general, behaviors and attitudes indicating that weight loss, dieting, and control of food are becoming primary concerns.

Health Consequences of Anorexia Nervosa:
- Anorexia Nervosa involves self-starvation. The body is denied the essential nutrients it needs to function normally, so it is forced to slow down all of its processes to conserve energy. This "slowing down" can have serious medical consequences:
- Abnormally slow heart rate and low blood pressure, which mean that the heart muscle is changing. The risk for heart failure rises as heart rate and blood pressure levels sink lower and lower.
- Reduction of bone density (osteoporosis), which results in dry, brittle bones.
- Muscle loss and weakness.
- Severe dehydration, which can result in kidney failure.
- Fainting, fatigue, and overall weakness.
- Dry hair and skin, hair loss is common.
- Growth of a downy layer of hair called lanugo all over the body, including the face, in an effort to keep the body warm.

Where to Get Help:

If you or someone you know is struggling with an eating disorder, The National Eating Disorders Association (NEDA) provides information, access and assistance to a wide variety of treatment options.

- Call toll free, confidential Helpline at 1-800-931-2237
  http://www.nationaleatingdisorders.org

The information included in this appendix was found on the NEDA website as of Feb. 15, 2014

Other Books by Bettie Youngs Book Publishers

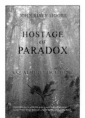

Hostage of Paradox: *A Qualmish Disclosure*

John Rixey Moore

Few people then or now know about the clandestine war that the CIA ran in Vietnam, using the Green Berets for secret operations throughout Southeast Asia. This was not the Vietnam War of the newsreels, the body counts, rice paddy footage, and men smoking cigarettes on the sandbag bunkers. This was a shadow directive of deep-penetration interdiction, reconnaissance, and assassination missions conducted by a selected few Special Forces units, deployed quietly from forward operations bases to prowl through agendas that, for security reasons, were seldom understood by the men themselves.

Hostage of Paradox is the first-hand account by one of these elite team leaders.

"Deserving of a place in the upper ranks of Vietnam War memoirs." —**Kirkus Review**

"Read this book, you'll be, as John Moore puts it, 'transfixed, like kittens in a box.'"
—**David Willson, Book Review, The VVA Veteran**

ISBN: 978-1-936332-37-3 • ePub: 978-1-936332-33-5

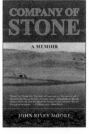

Company of Stone

John Rixey Moore

With yet unhealed wounds from recent combat, John Moore undertook an unexpected walking tour in the rugged Scottish highlands. With the approach of a season of freezing rainstorms he took shelter in a remote monastery—a chance encounter that would change his future, his beliefs about blind chance, and the unexpected courses by which the best in human nature can smuggle its way into the life of a stranger. Afterwards, a chance conversation overheard in a village pub steered him to Canada, where he took a job as a rock drill operator in a large industrial gold mine. The dangers he encountered among the lost men in that dangerous other world, secretive men who sought permanent anonymity in the perils of work deep underground—a brutal kind of monasticism itself—challenged both his endurance and his sense of humanity.

With sensitivity and delightful good humor, Moore explores the surprising lessons learned in these strangely rich fraternities of forgotten men—a brotherhood housed in crumbling medieval masonry, and one shared in the unforgiving depths of the gold mine.

ISBN: 978-1-936332-44-1 • ePub: 978-1-936332-45-8

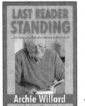

Last Reader Standing
... The Story of a Man Who Learned to Read at 54

Archie Willard
with Colleen Wiemerslage

The day Archie lost his thirty-one year job as a laborer at a meat packing company, he was forced to confront the secret he had held so closely for most of his life: at the age of fifty-four, he couldn't read. For all his adult life, he'd been able to skirt around the issue. But now, forced to find a new job to support his family, he could no longer hide from the truth.

Last Reader Standing is the story of Archie's amazing—and often painful—journey of becoming literate at middle age, struggling with the newfound knowledge of his dyslexia. From the little boy who was banished to the back of the classroom because the teachers labeled him "stupid," Archie emerged to becoming a national figure who continues to enlighten professionals into the world of the learning disabled. He joined Barbara Bush on stage for her Literacy Foundation's fundraisers where she proudly introduced him as "the man who took advantage of a second chance and improved his life."

This is a touching and poignant story that gives us an eye-opening view of the lack of literacy in our society, and how important it is for all of us to have opportunity to become all that we can be—to have hope and go after our dreams.

At the age of eighty-two, Archie continues to work with literacy issues in medicine and consumerism.

"Archie . . . you need to continue spreading the word." —**Barbara Bush, founder of the Literacy Foundation, and First Lady and wife of George H. W. Bush, the 41st President of the United States**

ISBN: 978-1-936332-48-9 • ePub: 978-1-936332-50-2

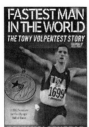

Fastest Man in the World
The Tony Volpentest Story

Tony Volpentest
Foreword by Ross Perot

Tony Volpentest, a four-time Paralympic gold medalist and five-time world champion sprinter, is a 2012 nominee for the Olympic Hall of Fame. This inspirational story details his being born without feet, to holding records as the fastest sprinter in the world.

"This inspiring story is about the thrill of victory to be sure—winning gold—but it is also a reminder about human potential: the willingness to push ourselves beyond the ledge of our own imagination. A powerfully inspirational story." —**Charlie Huebner, United States Olympic Committee**

ISBN: 978-1-940784-07-6 • ePub: 978-1-940784-08-3

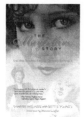

The Maybelline Story
And the Spirited Family Dynasty Behind It

Sharrie Williams

A fascinating and inspiring story, a tale both epic and intimate, alive with the clash, the hustle, the music, and dance of American enterprise.

"A richly told story of a forty-year, white-hot love triangle that fans the flames of a major worldwide conglomerate." —**Neil Shulman, Associate Producer,** *Doc Hollywood*

"Salacious! Engrossing! There are certain stories so dramatic, so sordid, that they seem positively destined for film; this is one of them." —*New York Post*

ISBN: 978-0-9843081-1-8 • ePub: 978-1-936332-17-5

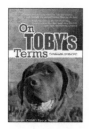

On Toby's Terms

Charmaine Hammond

On Toby's Terms is an endearing story of a beguiling creature who teaches his owners that, despite their trying to teach him how to be the dog they want, he is the one to lay out the terms of being the dog he needs to be. This insight would change their lives forever.

"This is a captivating, heartwarming story and we are very excited about bringing it to film." —**Steve Hudis, Producer**

ISBN: 978-0-9843081-4-9 • ePub: 978-1-936332-15-1

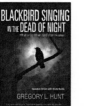

Blackbird Singing in the Dead of Night
What to Do When God Won't Answer

Updated Edition with Study Guide

Gregory L. Hunt

Pastor Greg Hunt had devoted nearly thirty years to congregational ministry, helping people experience God and find their way in life. Then came his own crisis of faith and calling. While turning to God for guidance, he finds nothing. Neither his education nor his religious involvements could prepare him for the disorienting impact of the experience. Alarmed, he tries an experiment. The result is startling—and changes his life entirely.

"Compelling. If you have ever longed to hear God whispering a love song into your life, read this book." —**Gary Chapman,** *NY Times* **bestselling author,** *The Love Languages of God*

ISBN: 978-0-9882848-9-0 • ePub: 978-1-936332-52-6

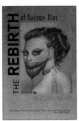

The Rebirth of Suzzan Blac

Suzzan Blac

A horrific upbringing and then abduction into the sex slave industry would all but kill Suzzan's spirit to live. But a happy marriage and two children brought love—and forty-two stunning paintings, art so raw that it initially frightened even the artist. "I hid the pieces for 15 years," says Suzzan, "but just as with the secrets in this book, I am slowing sneaking them out, one by one by one." Now a renowned artist, her work is exhibited world-wide. A story of inspiration, truth and victory.

"A solid memoir about a life reconstructed. Chilling, thrilling, and thought provoking."
—**Pearry Teo, Producer,** *The Gene Generation*

ISBN: 978-1-936332-22-9 • ePub: 978-1-936332-23-6

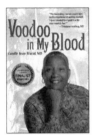

Voodoo in My Blood
A Healer's Journey from Surgeon to Shaman

Carolle Jean-Murat, M.D.

Born and raised in Haiti to a family of healers, US trained physician Carolle Jean-Murat came to be regarded as a world-class surgeon. But her success harbored a secret: in the operating room, she could quickly intuit the root cause of her patient's illness, often times knowing she could help the patient without surgery. Carolle knew that to fellow surgeons, her intuition was best left unmentioned. But when the devastating earthquake hit Haiti and Carolle returned to help, she had to acknowledge the shaman she had become.

"This fascinating memoir sheds light on the importance of asking yourself, 'Have I created for myself the life I've meant to live?'" —**Christiane Northrup, M.D., author of the New York Times bestsellers:** *Women's Bodies, Women's Wisdom*

ISBN: 978-1-936332-05-2 • ePub: 978-1-936332-04-5

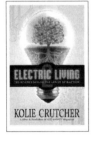

Electric Living
The Science behind the Law of Attraction

Kolie Crutcher

An electrical engineer by training, Crutcher applies his in-depth knowledge of electrical engineering principles and practical engineering experience detailing the scientific explanation of why human beings become what they think. A practical, step-by-step guide to help you harness your thoughts and emotions so that the Law of Attraction will benefit you.

ISBN: 978-1-936332-58-8 • ePub: 978-1-936332-59-5

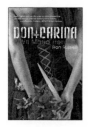

DON CARINA: *WWII Mafia Heroine*

Ron Russell

A father's death in Southern Italy in the 1930s—a place where women who can read are considered unfit for marriage—thrusts seventeen-year-old Carina into servitude as a "black widow," a legal head of the household who cares for her twelve siblings. A scandal forces her into a marriage to Russo, the "Prince of Naples." By cunning force, Carina seizes control of Russo's organization and disguising herself as a man, controls the most powerful of Mafia groups for nearly a decade.

"A woman as the head of the Mafia who shows her family her resourcefulness, strength and survival techniques. Unique, creative and powerful! This exciting book blends history, intrigue and power into one delicious epic adventure that you will not want to put down!" **—Linda Gray, Actress, *Dallas***

ISBN: 978-0-9843081-9-4 • ePub: 978-1-936332-49-6

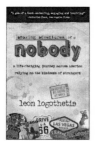

Amazing Adventures of a Nobody

Leon Logothetis

From the Hit Television Series Aired in 100 Countries!

Tired of his disconnected life and uninspiring job, Leon Logothetis leaves it all behind—job, money, home, even his cell phone—and hits the road with nothing but the clothes on his back and five dollars in his pocket, relying on the kindness of strangers and the serendipity of the open road for his daily keep. Masterful story-telling!

"A gem of a book; endearing, engaging and inspiring." **—Catharine Hamm, Los Angeles Times Travel Editor**

ISBN: 978-0-9843081-3-2 • ePub: 978-1-936332-51-9

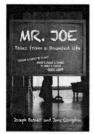

MR. JOE
Tales from a Haunted Life

Joseph Barnett and Jane Congdon

Do you believe in ghosts? Joseph Barnett didn't, until the winter he was fired from his career job and became a school custodian. Assigned the graveyard shift, Joe was confronted with a series of bizarre and terrifying occurrences.

"Thrilling, thoughtful, elegantly told. So much more than a ghost story." **—Cyrus Webb, CEO, Conversation Book Club**

ISBN: 978-1-936332-78-6 • ePub: 978-1-936332-79-3

Out of the Transylvania Night

Aura Imbarus
A Pulitzer-Prize entry

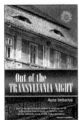

"I'd grown up in the land of Transylvania, homeland to Dracula, Vlad the Impaler, and worse, dictator Nicolae Ceausescu," writes the author. "Under his rule, like vampires, we came to life after sundown, hiding our heirloom jewels and documents deep in the earth." Fleeing to the US to rebuild her life, she discovers a startling truth about straddling two cultures and striking a balance between one's dreams and the sacrifices that allow a sense of "home."

"Aura's courage shows the degree to which we are all willing to live lives centered on freedom, hope, and an authentic sense of self. Truly a love story!" —**Nadia Comaneci, Olympic Champion**

ISBN: 978-0-9843081-2-5 • ePub: 978-1-936332-20-5

Living with Multiple Personalities
The Christine Ducommun Story

Christine Ducommun

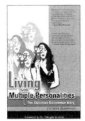

Christine Ducommun was a happily married wife and mother of two, when—after moving back into her childhood home—she began to experience panic attacks and bizarre flashbacks. Eventually diagnosed with Dissociative Identity Disorder (DID), Christine's story details an extraordinary twelve-year ordeal unraveling the buried trauma of her forgotten past.

"Reminiscent of the Academy Award-winning *A Beautiful Mind*, this true story will have you on the edge of your seat. Spellbinding!" —**Josh Miller, Producer**

ISBN: 978-0-9843081-5-6 • ePub: 978-1-936332-06-9

The Tortoise Shell Code

V Frank Asaro

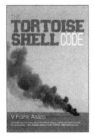

Off the coast of Southern California, the Sea Diva, a tuna boat, sinks. Members of the crew are missing and what happened remains a mystery. Anthony Darren, a renowned and wealthy lawyer at the top of his game, knows the boat's owner and soon becomes involved in the case. As the case goes to trial, a missing crew member is believed to be at fault, but new evidence comes to light and the finger of guilt points in a completely unanticipated direction. An action-packed thriller.

ISBN: 978-1-936332-60-1 • ePub: 978-1-936332-61-8

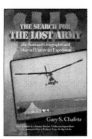

The Search for the Lost Army
The National Geographic and
Harvard University Expedition

Gary S. Chafetz

In one of history's greatest ancient disasters, a Persian army of 50,000 soldiers was suffocated by a hurricane-force sandstorm in 525 BC in Egypt's Western Desert. No trace of this conquering army, hauling huge quantities of looted gold and silver, has ever surfaced.

Gary Chafetz, referred to as "one of the ten best journalists of the past twenty-five years," is a former Boston Globe correspondent and was twice nominated for a Pulitzer Prize by the Globe.

ISBN: 978-1-936332-98-4 • ePub: 978-1-936332-99-1

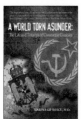

A World Torn Asunder
The Life and Triumph of Constantin C. Giurescu

Marina Giurescu, M.D.

Constantin C. Giurescu was Romania's leading historian and author. His granddaughter's fascinating story of this remarkable man and his family follows their struggles in war-torn Romania from 1900 to the fall of the Soviet Union. An "enlightened" society is dismantled with the 1946 Communist takeover of Romania, and Constantin is confined to the notorious Sighet penitentiary. Drawing on her grandfather's prison diary (which was put in a glass jar, buried in a yard, then smuggled out of the country by Dr. Paul E. Michelson—who does the FOREWORD for this book), private letters and her own research, Dr. Giurescu writes of the legacy from the turn of the century to the fall of Communism.

We see the rise of modern Romania, the misery of World War I, the blossoming of its culture between the wars, and then the sellout of Eastern Europe to Russia after World War II. In this sweeping account, we see not only its effects socially and culturally, but the triumph in its wake: a man and his people who reclaim better lives for themselves, and in the process, teach us a lesson in endurance, patience, and will—not only to survive, but to thrive.

"The inspirational story of a quiet man and his silent defiance in the face of tyranny."
—Dr. Connie Mariano, author of *The White House Doctor*

ISBN: 978-1-936332-76-2 • ePub: 978-1-936332-77-9

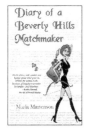

Diary of a Beverly Hills Matchmaker

Marla Martenson

Quick-witted Marla takes her readers for a hilarious romp through her days as an LA matchmaker where looks are everything and money talks. The Cupid of Beverly Hills has introduced countless couples who lived happily ever-after, but for every success story there are hysterically funny dating disasters with high-maintenance, out of touch clients. Marla writes with charm and self-effacement about the universal struggle to love and be loved.

ISBN 978-0-9843081-0-1 • ePub: 978-1-936332-03-8

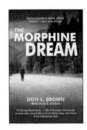

The Morphine Dream

Don Brown with Pulitzer nominated Gary S. Chafetz

At 36, high-school dropout and a failed semi-professional ballplayer Donald Brown hit bottom when an industrial accident left him immobilized. But Brown had a dream while on a morphine drip after surgery: he imagined himself graduating from Harvard Law School (he was a classmate of Barack Obama) and walking across America. Brown realizes both seemingly unreachable goals, and achieves national recognition as a legal crusader for minority homeowners. An intriguing tale of his long walk—both physical and metaphorical. A story of perseverance and second chances. Sheer inspiration for those wishing to reboot their lives.

"An incredibly inspirational memoir." —Alan M. Dershowitz, professor, Harvard Law School

ISBN: 978-1-936332-25-0 • ePub: 978-1-936332-39-7

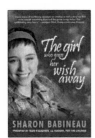

The Girl Who Gave Her Wish Away

Sharon Babineau
Foreword by Craig Kielburger

The Children's Wish Foundation approached lovely thirteen-year-old Maddison Babineau just after she received her cancer diagnosis. "You can have anything," they told her, "a Disney cruise? The chance to meet your favorite movie star? A five thousand dollar shopping spree?"

Maddie knew exactly what she wanted. She had recently been moved to tears after watching a television program about the plight of orphaned children. Maddie's wish? To ease the suffering of these children half-way across the world. Despite the ravishing cancer, she became an indefatigable fundraiser for "her children." In The Girl Who Gave Wish Away, her mother reveals Maddie's remarkable journey of providing hope and future to the village children who had filled her heart.

A special story, heartwarming and reassuring.

ISBN: 978-1-936332-96-0 • ePub: 978-1-936332-97-7

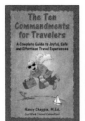

The Ten Commandments for Travelers

Nancy Chappie

Traveling can be an overwhelming experience fraught with delays, tension, and unexpected complications. But whether you're traveling for business or pleasure, alone or with family or friends, there are things you can do to make your travels more enjoyable—even during the most challenging experiences. Easy to implement tips for hassle-free travel, and guidance for those moments that threaten to turn your voyage into an unpleasant experience. You'll learn how to avoid extra costs and aggravations, save time, and stay safe; how to keep your cool under the worst of circumstances, how to embrace new cultures, and how to fully enjoy each moment you're on the road.

ISBN: 978-1-936332-74-8 • ePub: 978-1-936332-75-5

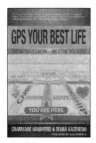

GPS YOUR BEST LIFE
Charting Your Destination and Getting There in Style

Charmaine Hammond and Debra Kasowski
Foreword by Jack Canfield

A most useful guide to charting and traversing the many options that lay before you.

"A perfect book for servicing your most important vehicle: yourself. No matter where you are in your life, the concepts and direction provided in this book will help you get to a better place. It's a must read." —**Ken Kragen, author of** *Life Is a Contact Sport*, **and organizer of** *We Are the World*, **and** *Hands Across America*, **and other historic humanitarian events**

ISBN: 978-1-936332-26-7 • ePub: 978-1-936332-41-0

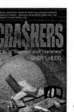

Crashers
A Tale of "Cappers" and "Hammers"

Lindy S. Hudis

The illegal business of fraudulent car accidents is a multi-million dollar racket, involving unscrupulous medical providers, personal injury attorneys, and the cooperating passengers involved in the accidents. Innocent people are often swept into it. Newly engaged Nathan and Shari, who are swimming in mounting debt, were easy prey: seduced by an offer from a stranger to move from hard times to good times in no time, Shari finds herself the "victim" in a staged auto accident. Shari gets her payday, but breaking free of this dark underworld will take nothing short of a miracle.

"A riveting story of love, life—and limits. A non-stop thrill ride." —**Dennis "Danger" Madalone, stunt coordinator,** *Castle*

ISBN: 978-1-936332-27-4 • ePub: 978-1-936332-28-1

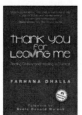

Thank You for Leaving Me
Finding Divinity and Healing in Divorce

Farhana Dhalla
Foreword by Neale Donald Walsch

The end of any relationship, especially divorce, can leave us bereft, feeling unmoored, empty. Speaking to that part of our hearts that knows you must find your way to a new and different place, this compassionate book of words of wisdom helps grow this glimmering knowledge—and offers hope and healing for turning this painful time into one of renewal and rediscovery. This book is balm for your wounded heart, and can help you turn your fragility to endurable coping, and will you rediscover your inner strengths. Best of all, this book will help you realize the transformative power inherent in this transition.

ISBN: 978-1-936332-85-4 • ePub: 978-1-936332-86-1

Truth Never Dies

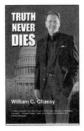

William C. Chasey

A lobbyist for some 40 years, William C. Chasey represented some of the world's most prestigious business clients and twenty-three foreign governments before the US Congress. His integrity never questioned. All that changed when Chasey was hired to forge communications between Libya and the US Congress. A trip he took with a US Congressman for discussions with then Libyan leader Muammar Qadhafi forever changed Chasey's life. Upon his return, his bank accounts were frozen, clients and friends had been advised not to take his calls.

Things got worse: the CIA, FBI, IRS, and the Federal Judiciary attempted to coerce him into using his unique Libyan access to participate in a CIA-sponsored assassination plot of the two Libyans indicted for the bombing of Pan Am flight 103. Chasey's refusal to cooperate resulted in a six-year FBI investigation and sting operation, financial ruin, criminal charges, and incarceration in federal prison.

ISBN: 978-1-936332-46-5 • ePub: 978-1-936332-47-2

Trafficking the Good Life

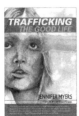

Jennifer Myers

Jennifer Myers had worked hard toward a successful career as a dancer in Chicago. But just as her star was rising, she fell for the kingpin of a drug trafficking operation. Drawn to his life of excitement, she soon acquiesced to driving marijuana across the country, making easy money she stacked in shoeboxes and spent like an heiress. Only time in a federal prison made her face up to and understand her choices. It was there, at rock bottom, that she discovered that her real prison was the one she had unwittingly made inside herself and where she could start rebuilding a life of purpose and ethical pursuit.

"In her gripping memoir Jennifer Myers offers a startling account of how the pursuit of an elusive American Dream can lead us to the depths of the American criminal underbelly. Her book is as much about being human in a hyper-materialistic society as it is about drug culture. When the DEA finally knocks on Myers' door, she and the reader both see the moment for what it truly is—not so much an arrest as a rescue." —**Tony D'Souza, author of Whiteman and Mule**

ISBN: 978-1-936332-67-0 • ePub: 978-1-936332-68-7

Universal Co-opetition
Nature's Fusion of Co-operation and Competition

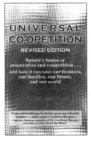

V Frank Asaro

A key ingredient in personal and business success is competition—and cooperation. Too much of one or the other can erode personal and organizational goals. This book identifies and explains the natural, fundamental law that unifies the apparently opposing forces of cooperation and competition.

ISBN: 978-1-936332-08-3 • ePub: 978-1-936332-09-0